The HealthMark Program for Life

The HealthMark Program for Life

BY

ROBERT A. GLESER, M.D.

McGRAW-HILL BOOK COMPANY
New York   St. Louis   San Francisco
Hamburg   Mexico   Toronto

Even though the author believes the information in this book to be as complete, accurate, and up-to-date as possible, any application of the recommendations set forth in the following pages is at the reader's discretion and risk. This book is not intended to replace the services of a physician, who should be consulted regarding any medical questions you may have.

1 2 3 4 5 6 7 8 9 DOC DOC 8 9 2 1 0 9 8

ISBN 0-07-023494-9

Library of Congress Cataloging-in-Publication Data

Gleser, Robert A.
  The HealthMark program for life / by Robert A. Gleser.
    p. cm.
  Includes index.
  ISBN 0-07-023494-9
  1. Health.   2. Nutrition.   3. Exercise—Health aspects.
  I. Title.
  RA776.G57   1988   88-9125
  613—dc19   CIP

Book design by Eve Kirch

To my late father, Issy. If I'd known then what I know now. . . .

To Denise, Dani, Ramon, and Ellie for your patience, perseverance, and sacrifice in helping me live my dreams.

To the thousands of HealthMark graduates who have made the change.

Contents

Preface

WHY THE HEALTHMARK PROGRAM?

Flirting with self-destruction has always been a romantic notion. We enjoy the dangers and thrill of speed, height, and endurance ...the thrill of victory and the agony of defeat. But when we consciously or unconsciously cause our self-destruction by damaging our health, there is no thrill of victory, only the agony of defeat.

The health status of most Americans today can be likened to a runaway train. We are totally out of control, eating the wrong foods, exercising too little, smoking and drinking too much. The train (our health) will eventually run into a disaster, which in terms of annual deaths may look like this:

1. Heart attacks—550,000

2. Stroke—170,000

3. Diabetes, adult-onset—136,000

4. Lung cancer—130,000

5. Colon cancer—60,000

6. Breast cancer—40,000

7. Prostate cancer—26,000

Moreover, 58 million people are affected by high blood pressure. These eight diseases account for almost 65 percent of all deaths and are for the most part preventable.

If we stop smoking, the majority of lung cancers will disappear. If we reduce our intake of fat and cholesterol and eat more fiber, the incidence of the other seven diseases will be reduced drastically, because these diseases are related to nutrition. It is as simple as learning to eat correctly, exercise safely, stop smoking, and reduce alcohol intake. By gaining control of controllable risks, we can certainly improve the quality of our lives and probably lengthen them as well.

The changes are simple and easy to make. Fear of making the change is our biggest stumbling block. When we realize that the "good things" we are so afraid to give up are actually the seeds of our own destruction, the choice becomes easy.

Unfortunately, the motivation to change lifestyle is usually an actual or impending disaster. In my case it was no different. There is a strong history of heart disease in my family, and I knew that I would some day have to make some change. By the age of 33 I had been only partially successful with the effort to change my habits. A bout with cancer really woke me up. I had always exercised regularly and had given up smoking 3 years previously, but my eating habits still left a lot to be desired. I had testicular cancer (a young man's cancer), and it took two operations to make sure everything was all right. The second operation was a 6-hour affair. I sailed through it because I was in reasonably good health. No further therapy was required (radiation or chemotherapy). Fortunately I am here 9½ years later, obviously thankful.

I am a physician—an internist and cancer therapist by training, and I was fully aware of the consequences of my lifestyle. Yet it took a life-threatening event to motivate me to make the change. No, my disease was not cured by diet and exercise but by good surgeons.

My interest in preventive medicine was sparked by this event. After making necessary dietary changes, I began to experience what "feeling good" really meant. You develop a glow and begin to feel that your body is functioning like a well-oiled machine. When you do eat a "bad" meal, somehow your body does not function as well—you feel like you have been run over by a truck! On this HealthMark program you are allowed what I call "10 percent time," or time for cheats and treats. Amazingly, after a few months you will notice that your body becomes less tolerant of the abuse and the desire to cheat becomes less and less.

After 2 years of practicing preventive medicine within the confines of my private practice, I decided to pursue this speciality full time. It was very difficult and frustrating to practice preventive medicine on my own because I needed the support of nutritionists, exercise physiologists, and psychologists to provide the necessary education. This realization finally led me to the Pritikin Longevity Center in Santa Monica, California, where I was the medical director from 1980 to 1982. I subsequently returned to Colorado and set up the HealthMark program in 1984. In the last 3 years more than 4000 participants have graduated from Health-Mark. My experience in preventive medicine over the last 9 years can best be described as a medical wonderland. Most traditional medical professionals would have difficulty comprehending the fascinating changes I have seen simply by lowering cholesterol, fat, salt, and alcohol intake; stopping smoking; losing weight; and exercising.

An important phenomenon occurs in people who make the lifestyle change. They tell you that they have not felt so well in years. Regaining control and responsibility for your health and steadily improving your body image, self-esteem, and confidence make you feel wonderful. However, I constantly hear the comment, "I feel good. Why should I make any changes?" Feeling "good" is relative, and only by making the necessary changes can you appreciate how good you can really feel. Why would you not want to feel well, or, if you have made the change, why would you not want to continue these good feelings? This is the motivation to make the changes and to continue with them. *Living long and healthy is too easy to pass up.*

The changes you can expect with the HealthMark program are listed below. They are what we have come to regard as routine and are based on the experience of more than 4000 people who have gone through the HealthMark programs in Denver, Colorado, in the past 3 years.

1. You feel good. Many graduates of our programs tell us, "I have not felt this good in years." Your self-esteem and ego get a real boost from the healthy feeling you experience, and nothing is more motivating to keep you on track. Most people do not want to go back to feeling bad.

2. You regain control. It is great knowing that you can be in control of the factors that influence your present and future health. We all want to guide our own destiny.

3. You can eat more and yet still lose weight. Some Health-Mark participants have lost 100 pounds or more. Our aim is slow and steady. In 3 weeks men on an average lose 6 to 10 pounds and women 4 to 6 pounds.

4. Cholesterol levels will drop an average of 20 to 25 percent in 3 weeks and normalize within a few months. Some people's cholesterol levels have dropped over 100 milligrams in 3 weeks. If cholesterol levels do not change appreciably and are still elevated after 6 months, then medication is used in conjunction with the diet. Elevated triglycerides also drop dramatically.

5. Coronary heart disease patients with angina and patients with postcoronary bypass do excellently. Angina pains soon disappear, and these patients rely less on medication to relieve the pain. Improved exercise tolerance and confidence in their own abilities, as well as the realization that this therapy is really something beneficial and specific to treat cholesterol buildup in arteries, gives patients a great psychological boost. The HealthMark program is a far better and less dangerous alternative to bypass and other surgical procedures.

   A few patients had abnormal treadmill stress tests initially (indicating the presence of probable coronary artery disease). They normalized their treadmill tests within 1 to 2 years by following the HealthMark program and reducing their coronary risk factors. We assume that this indicates a reversal in the cholesterol blockages that caused the original electrocardiogram abnormalities.

6. Peripheral vascular disease is attributed to cholesterol blockages in the legs that cause pain when walking. After a few weeks of low fat, low cholesterol food and exercise, people often find that their leg pain diminishes and may eventually disappear. We have had participants in our program who originally could not walk very far without pain who now are walking 2 to 3 miles per day after 3 to 4 weeks.

7. High blood pressure melts away rapidly. Within 1 to 2 weeks most people don't need their medication, and it is tapered and discontinued where appropriate.

8. Adult-onset diabetes also resolves rapidly and dramatically. We have graduates who are off insulin and oral medication and are living normal lives.

9. Heartburn and ulcer pains respond dramatically.

10. Symptoms of degenerative arthritis improve with weight loss and muscle strengthening around joints. We have had a few people who have showed improvements in rheumatoid arthritis. We don't know the reason for this improvement.

11. Elderly people do wonderfully. Getting them mobilized and active as well as eating healthy food produces some wonderful changes and many times gives them new outlooks on life.

A program for change works only if it produces long-term results. Many dietary programs are so restrictive (8 to 10 percent of total calories as fat) that they are difficult to adhere to. These programs produce good short-term results, but when you fail in 6 to 8 weeks, the rebound (overeating, smoking, and drinking) may put you in worse shape than when you began. However, a program that is too liberal (30 percent fat) will not produce the desired changes.

The HealthMark program (20 percent fat) is designed to be middle of the road. The restrictions are sufficient to produce the necessary changes, yet you can have familiar-looking, palatable foods.

When we look at end results such as cholesterol and triglyceride (fat) levels in the blood, the decreases achieved at the end of 3 to 4 weeks on a 20 percent or an 8 to 10 percent fat diet are the same. Therefore, there is no need to restrict yourself unnecessarily. Why eat steamed vegetables for the rest of your life when you can enjoy the variety of eating fish, chicken, and low fat beef (all the foods you are used to eating), if prepared the correct way?

In addition, you need to set other goals to succeed—goals for weight, blood cholesterol, triglycerides, blood sugar levels, blood pressure, and for monitoring symptoms of cardiovascular disease and diabetes.

Finally, there needs to be a balance among nutrition, exercise, and stress management for optimal results.

Acknowledgments

I would like to acknowledge the late Nathan Pritikin, whose teachings and inspiration had an enormous impact on my life. This book owes its existence to the many people with whom I work and who have had a hand in helping me develop HealthMark into a unique, outstanding, and innovative preventive medicine program and clinic.

I would like to thank HealthMark's director of nutrition, Susan Stevens, M.S., R.D., and Robin Purnell, R.D., for their help in developing the recipes and diet plans presented here; HealthMark's director of exercise physiology, Mary Schneider, M.S., for her help with the exercise section; and Dr. Wayne Peters, whose academic knowledge has been invaluable throughout the preparation of this book. I would also like to thank Joel Janco, Kathy Walker, Coleen Custy, and all the energetic HealthMark staff for their contributions to the success of HealthMark; Ira Gleser and Jacqui Grusd for their continuing love and support; Barbara Tanton for her fine typing; and Tom Quinn and Ann Craig for their patient editing. And finally, I would like to thank the 128 Safeway and Toddy's supermarkets in the Rocky Mountain region who have HealthMarked the thousands of healthy foods on their shelves and the more than 100 restaurants in the Denver region who have provided Health-Mark-approved items on their menus and showed that health food can look appetizing and taste great.

Introduction

WHY SHOULD WE MAKE THE CHANGE?

The evidence is clear that there is a strong relationship between our eating, drinking, and smoking habits, our lack of exercise, and the leading causes of death. Additionally, there are a host of less-threatening diseases that appear to be nutrition-related. These include gallstones, obesity, degenerative arthritis, diverticulosis, spastic colon, venous thrombosis, hiatal hernia, and constipation.

In various third world cultures where people eat low fat, low cholesterol, high fiber foods and lead active unstressed lives, these diseases are nonexistent or occur much less frequently than in the Western world. Many great cultures have been built on complex carbohydrates (rice, beans, corn, and potatoes).

Our ancestors (the cave dwellers) ate well. Their diet consisted of nuts, seeds, legumes (complex carbohydrates), and occasional lean meat. There were no feedlots to fatten their meat and no food-processing plants to refine their carbohydrates into white flour, sugar, and white rice. These ancestors were the hunters and gatherers, and yet they died very young from diseases that we can easily cure with drugs such as penicillin. Today we have a wide range of antibiotics and sophisticated medical technology, and our life span has increased (72.5 years for men and 78 for women). Our life span increased greatly after the discovery of antibiotics and has not in-

1

creased much since. We are probably close to the limit of life span that can be achieved with technology. The new frontier of preventive medicine should cause the next major increase in longevity through the prevention of cardiovascular disease, cancer, high blood pressure, and diabetes.

The cave dweller's genes we have inherited were not meant to protect us from the onslaught of fat, cholesterol, salt, alcohol, carbon monoxide, and nicotine (from smoking). Eventually our bodies break down with heart attacks, strokes, diabetes, high blood pressure, and cancer. It's like feeding your car bad fuel—it will break down.

HOW DO WE MAKE THE CHANGE?

Why don't we simply adopt the eating habits of the third world people such as the Tarahumara Indians of central Mexico or the people of Guinea? They eat 8 to 10 percent of their calories as fat, a tremendous amount of fiber, and fewer than 100 milligrams of cholesterol per day. Unfortunately, these people are not living in the "civilized world" and can neither afford nor find available the sources of food that we have. We in the Western world are living at the other extreme—overindulgence. It is impractical and unnecessary to expect us to adapt these extreme dietary habits or maintain them to achieve optimal health and longevity.

Table I-1 makes some dietary comparisons.

Table I-1   Average Daily Dietary Intake

	Typical U.S. Diet	HealthMark Diet	Third-World Diet
Cholesterol (mg)	450–750	150	50
Percentage of daily calories			
Fat	40	20	8–10
Protein	15–20	10–15	10–15
Carbohydrate	40–45	65	75–80

Extremely low fat diets (8 to 10 percent) are available and have been modeled on third-world eating habits. They are mostly unsuccessful because they cannot produce long-term compliance. Good short-term results are achieved, but failure usually occurs in 6 to 8 weeks. Scientific evidence has shown that the extremely low fat diets do not produce any greater decrease in cholesterol and triglyceride levels than do more moderate (20 percent fat) diets over a 3- to 4-week period.

Moderate diets with a balanced fat intake (such as the Health-Mark program) are geared to produce long-term compliance by providing a wider variety of familiar and palatable foods. In fact, on the HealthMark program you can eat all the foods you used to eat (with only a few exceptions); however, the foods are prepared differently. Long-term compliance is the key to success on any dietary program.

Every program needs a balanced approach. All three disciplines—nutrition, exercise, and stress management (self-management)—make up the basis of the HealthMark program. We need to develop practical, sensible, and easy ways to live.

Nutrition

A low fat, low cholesterol, and high fiber eating program is necessary. We must produce palatable and familiar food and avoid the syndrome of "if it's good for you, it must taste bland." The Health-Mark program allows you to use most of the foods you are accustomed to eating. The food looks familiar and tastes good.

Exercise

We don't need to become marathoners, triathletes, or olympians, but we should exercise regularly enough to maintain cardiovascular fitness.

Stress

We cannot be devoid of all stress. If you achieve this no-stress state, you will probably lose all your drive and ambition. A balance between positive and negative stress needs to be reached.

Where Does the Responsibility Lie?

The only person responsible for your health is you. It is up to you to find out what factors place you at risk and do something to modify them, e.g., cholesterol, blood pressure, triglycerides, and weight. Unfortunately, you cannot rely on most of the medical profession to advise you adequately on this, and you must assume the responsibility yourself. Doctors are geared toward treating acute illness and not prevention.

O N E

Playing Russian Roulette with Our Health

Living is risky business—like a game of Russian roulette. We need to become aware of the risk factors for the leading causes of death and disease and regard them as bullets in a gun. These risk factors are elevated cholesterol and other lipid abnormalities, high blood pressure, diabetes, smoking, obesity, high fat diets, lack of exercise, and chemical pollutants in food and the environment. These risk factors are as dangerous as real bullets. The more risk factors (bullets) in the gun, the greater the chances are of killing or maiming yourself.

Each of these risk factors is reversible, and reducing risk can be likened to removing bullets from the gun, thus increasing your chances at survival.

We don't ignore fire, flood, or tornado warnings. Why do we ignore warnings about our health? We need to develop awareness about how much we actually control our health.

CARDIOVASCULAR DISEASES

Common cardiovascular diseases are caused by cholesterol deposits in the arterial wall (atherosclerosis). Any artery in the body can be affected. The commonest occlusions are in the coronary arteries (heart attacks), cerebral arteries (strokes), and the arteries to the leg (peripheral vascular disease). Symptoms will not develop until the artery is blocked 70 percent or more.

Cardiovascular disease is the leading cause of death in the United States today. Nearly 25 percent of all adults have some form of cardiovascular disease. Indeed, 5 million Americans have documented coronary artery disease, and 1.25 million have heart attacks annually. *About 550,000 people die annually from heart attacks and in 30 percent of the people who develop coronary artery disease, the first symptom is sudden death,* obviously a scenario you wish to avoid. Having survived a heart attack or the development of angina, you still may be able to do a great deal to help yourself.

Coronary Artery Disease

The heart muscle is a pump and requires the oxygen delivered by the red blood cells. When this muscle is starved for oxygen, a pain called *angina* will result. A coronary artery blocked 60 to 70 percent may be able to deliver enough blood flow at rest to provide oxygen. As soon as the heart begins to beat faster, however, the amount of blood getting through the blockage will be insufficient to supply oxygen, and pain (or angina) will result. Exercise, eating heavy meals, stress, and cold weather are the usual factors causing your heart rate (or pulse) to rise, thereby precipitating angina.

Angina is usually felt as a left-sided chest pressure often traveling to the left arm. It is often described as a "vise around my chest, a heaviness in my chest, or a truck going back and forward over my chest." The pain may be felt occasionally as neck or jaw pain, wrist pain, back pain, or abdominal pain. It usually lasts 15 minutes or less and is relieved by rest. Pain that lasts longer than this may be from a heart attack and requires prompt attention by qualified medical personnel.

Complete blockage of a coronary artery will produce a heart attack in which the heart muscle affected actually dies and is replaced by scar tissue. If the damage is severe, the heart muscle will become an ineffective pump, and heart failure will result. The disability that results depends on the extent of damage and scarring incurred at the time of the heart attack, if the victim survives.

This information is meant to inform you, not to allow you to self-diagnose. Any chest pain that develops at rest or with exercise should be investigated by the appropriate medical personnel, particularly if it is a first-time occurrence. Only those people who have had recurrent angina and recognize the typical pains can observe them, providing the pains do not last longer than 15 minutes and do not increase in frequency or severity.

The bottom line is that if you develop chest pain, it needs to be investigated.

Medical treatment in cases of acute heart attack is a topic that lies outside the scope of this book. Heart attacks should be treated in hospitals, in coronary care units, by qualified cardiologists and other qualified medical professionals. Decisions regarding further management (coronary bypass or angioplasty) are based on the medical circumstances at the time and the advice of the team of professionals in charge of your care. These alternatives need to be explored if a life-threatening situation exists.

For the chronic management of coronary artery disease, two traditional forms of therapy exist: (1) medical and (2) surgical.

Medical Treatment for Coronary Artery Disease

Medications are prescribed to help relieve angina to make your daily functions easier. Nitroglycerin tablets taken under the tongue are effective in relieving pain. Additionally, there are medications that reduce the work load of the heart, thus reducing the frequency and severity of angina attacks. These medications are called *beta blockers* and *calcium channel blockers* and are available under a host of different trade names.

These medications are effective in what they do, i.e., relieve angina. Unfortunately, they do not tackle the underlying problem of cholesterol buildup in the arteries. It is negligent to take these medications and ignore treating the lipid disorder and other risk factors that must be present. In fact, some of these medications (specifically, beta blockers) can cause abnormalities in blood lipids, which is counterproductive. The decision to take these should be weighed against the magnitude of the lipid disorder; i.e., if you are able to control your lipids easily despite taking the medications, there is no problem. If you have trouble normalizing your lipid values, you need to consider changing the medication to something that does not raise them, if this change is medically feasible. Obviously, this must be done under the supervision of your physician.

Surgical Treatment for Coronary Artery Disease

Two generally accepted surgical procedures are available today.

1. *Balloon angioplasty:* A thin plastic catheter is passed through the blocked artery, and a balloon surrounding the catheter is inflated and squashes or flattens the cholesterol plaque, thus reopening the artery. This procedure is successful on isolated blockages; however, complications do occur which sometimes require emergency bypass surgery. There is also a significant incidence of restenosis (reblockage) within a few months of the procedure.

2. *Coronary bypass:* In coronary bypass procedures, the blocked arteries are bypassed with either veins stripped from the legs or a small artery taken from inside the chest wall (internal mammary). With vein bypass the veins are attached to the aorta (the main artery arising from the heart) and beyond the blockage. There are obvious potential complications from this procedure:

- A 1 to 2 percent operative mortality exists.

- In a small percentage of people blood clots may block the bypass in the first few months after surgery.

- Reoccurrence of atherosclerosis will occur in the new vein grafts as well as progression of the original blockages in the native vessels. A study in Montreal showed that 80 percent of the bypasses are blocked by cholesterol buildup within 8 years. The internal mammary grafts appear to remain open longer because the thicker-walled arteries appear to be more resistant to atherosclerosis than the thin-walled veins.

For the majority, the 5- and 10-year survival rates for standard medical or surgical therapy do not appear to differ. Thus the need for bypass should be greatly reduced. This does not mean that bypass should never be done; there are people who will benefit from it. People whose lives are threatened by severe blockages in all three coronary arteries or who have a blockage in the main left coronary artery need surgical intervention. A maximal treadmill test will usually show some changes very early on in the test, and this will be an indication to proceed with an angiogram and possibly bypass or angioplasty, as lifesaving measures.

Angioplasty is a relatively new procedure, and its exact role is currently being defined. Angioplasty can be performed only for isolated blockages that are relatively close to the mouth of the artery. This procedure is safer and much less expensive than bypass.

In summary, the benefits of bypass or angioplasty are specific in their lifesaving abilities. However, they do nothing to affect the actual process of atherosclerosis. Atherosclerosis will develop in the bypass or vessel opened by angioplasty and will progress in the original (native) coronary arteries if no risk factor modification is done.

Coronary bypass and angioplasty should never be performed without coronary risk factor modification as a routine part of the therapy management.

There is a third and more specific therapy for atherosclerosis called *risk factor modification*. Atherosclerosis is a multifactor disease. In our attempts to halt and reverse its progression, we need to attack the causes or risk factors in a balanced approach. It's as simple as the following list of goals:

Lower cholesterol below 160 mg.

Lower cholesterol-HDL ratio below 3.5.

Control blood pressure.

Stop smoking.

Control diabetes.

Lose weight.

Lower triglycerides.

Exercise regularly.

Reduce stress levels.

That's it. Crazy as it may appear, this is the most specific treatment for atherosclerosis (see reversing atherosclerosis, page 56). Therefore, the most specific treatment for heart disease is the least expensive and the most safe. It's called lifestyle change: learning to eat correctly, exercise regularly, and stop smoking. If we all do this, bypass operations, angioplasty, and even heart disease may become a thing of the past.

Stroke

The buildup of plaque (atherosclerosis) in the arteries to the head and neck will eventually cause strokes. A complete occlusion will cause a major stroke, with all of its devastating consequences, such as paralysis and speech impediments, usually with permanent disability.

Fragments of cholesterol plaque in the carotid arteries (the big arteries in the neck) can break off and cause minor strokes called *transient ischemic attacks* (TIAs). These strokes cause symptoms that last fewer than 24 hours and resolve without any residual defects. However, these are usually the forerunners of more serious strokes.

The TIAs should usually be treated with thinning of the blood and risk factor modification. Surgery to bypass the blockage or to ream out the artery (endarterectomy) is controversial. The hazards of the surgery (strokes) should be weighed against the possible benefits, and a conservative approach is usually indicated.

A major stroke should be treated with the appropriate rehabilitation and risk factor modification. A neurologist should determine the exact acute treatment based on whether the stroke was caused by hemorrhage (bleeding into the brain usually caused by high blood pressure) or a complete occlusion of the artery (usually caused by a blood clot on top of the cholesterol plaque).

Peripheral Vascular Disease

Plaque buildup in the main arteries to the legs will cause, with walking, pain in the calves and thighs, and the leg usually becomes pale and cold. The pain when walking is called *intermittent claudication*. Surgery with bypass and endarterectomy should only be considered for impending gangrene of the leg or foot. Dramatic improvements have been noticed with regular exercise, no smoking, and lowering lipids, i.e., risk factor modification. We have treated people who could not walk more than a few steps before feeling claudication. After a few months of risk factor modification, they are able to walk a few miles before getting some if any pain.

When angina occurs, exercise needs to be stopped immediately. When claudication occurs, however, you can try to walk through the pain and stop to rest when the pain becomes too severe. The lack of oxygen arising with claudication may be beneficial in inducing new blood vessels to grow (called *collaterals*) which bypass the blocked arteries. However, this practice is too dangerous with angina because the lack of oxygen to the heart muscle may cause heart attacks.

Never try to exercise through your angina or chest pain— always stop and rest.

Aneurysm

Aneurysm occurs when atherosclerosis causes a weakening of the arterial wall resulting in a ballooning or dilatation of the artery.

It may rupture and cause sudden death. Aneurysms always need to be treated by surgical repair, i.e., replacement of the diseased artery with a graft. This should be done on an elective basis by diagnosing it before the rupture, rather than trying to treat it as an emergency once rupture has occurred, since such rupture can be life-threatening.

Aneurysms that occur in the arteries in the brain are often congenital rather than atherosclerotic; i.e., they are caused by congenital weaknesses rather than cholesterol buildup and should be treated surgically whenever feasible.

HIGH BLOOD PRESSURE (HYPERTENSION)

Approximately 58 million adults in the United States have high blood pressure (HBP). One in three adults have it, many unknowingly. HBP is called the "silent killer." Sustained elevation of the blood pressure will cause heart attacks, strokes, and kidney failure.

The upper limits of normal are defined as any readings below 140/90 millimeters of mercury (mm Hg). Ideally, blood pressure readings should be at 100 to 120/60 to 80 mm Hg or less. The heart is continually contracting and relaxing as it works as a pump to squeeze blood into the blood vessels. The upper reading, or *systolic*, reflects the pressure in the arteries during the heart's contraction phase. The lower reading, or *diastolic*, reflects the pressure in the arteries during the heart's relaxation phase. The diastolic blood pressure reflects the resistance in the peripheral arteries that may be elevated by narrowing (spasm), or if there is too much fluid in the system (blood vessels), e.g., the water retention that occurs with salt ingestion.

Mild elevations of blood pressure are responsible for almost half the deaths attributed to HBP. The common line, "Your pressure is mildly elevated—don't worry about it," is reason for concern. If you have your blood pressure checked once in a while and find that it is mildly elevated, you must act. The first thing to do is buy a blood pressure cuff and monitor your pressure daily. If your blood pressure is elevated regularly, then it needs to be treated. Isolated elevated blood pressure readings are not meaningful—your pressure needs to be elevated on three or more occasions to qualify as high blood pressure.

Many studies have shown that treatment of HBP will prevent medical complications, especially strokes. There are two methods of treatment available: (1) medication and (2) diet and exercise.

Medication in the Treatment of High Blood Pressure

A host of medication exists that can effectively control HBP; however, there are always the problems of compliance and side effects.

Studies using medication to treat blood pressure have shown that the risk of stroke is greatly reduced. The risk for heart attack, however, may be elevated in these same individuals, possibly because many blood pressure medications used today actually elevate cholesterol or triglycerides. When taking medications, be sure your medicine does not have this potential. A variety of drugs that are good for treating blood pressure don't affect lipid values (see Table 1-1).

Ask your physician about your medication for blood pressure and whether it should be changed.

Diet and Exercise in the Treatment of High Blood Pressure

A host of nutritional, stress, and exercise factors are responsible for HBP. Reversing these factors normalizes blood pressure in most people.

1. *Exercise:* Chronic, sustained aerobic exercise is probably one of the best methods to treat HBP. Exercise causes the release of naturally occurring tranquilizing hormones (endorphins), which relax you and help lower blood pressure. In addition, exercise will cause relaxation, or dilatation, of the arteries, which will lower blood pressure. Exercise will also result in weight loss, helping to lower blood pressure.

Table 1-1   Effects of Selected Drugs on Lipid Levels

Drug	Total Cholesterol	HDL[1]	Triglyceride
Thiazide diuretics	I[2]	—[3]	—
Aldactone/spironolactone	I	—	I
Beta blockers	—	D[4]	I
Calcium channel blockers	—	—	—
ACE inhibitors	—	—	—
Vasodilators	D	I	—
Zyloprim (for gout)	—	—	I

[1] *"Good" cholesterol. (See Chapter Two.)*

[2] *I: Increases.*

[3] *—: No effect.*

[4] *D: Decreases.*

2. *Obesity:* There is a direct relationship between obesity and HBP. Weight loss lowers blood pressure regardless of changes in other causes.

3. *Salt (sodium chloride):* We eat 3 to 5 teaspoons of salt per day in the United States and need only 1 teaspoon per day. One teaspoon contains 2300 milligrams of sodium. Sodium causes the retention of fluid (we get thirsty when we eat salt), and the resultant expansion of the blood volume will cause HBP. A reduction in sodium intake causes the excess sodium to pass out of the kidneys, taking with it all the excess fluid. You will notice that you pass urine more often until all the excess sodium and fluid is removed. This is how a diuretic (water pill) works. Not everyone is salt-sensitive, however, but most people with HBP are, and thus they need to restrict sodium intake.

4. *Potassium:* A low potassium intake or a low blood potassium level is related to HBP. A high salt diet will make

you lose potassium in the urine as the kidneys exchange sodium for potassium. In addition, diuretics usually cause a loss of potassium in the urine, and this may aggravate HBP. Diuretics are not a good choice, therefore, for the treatment of HBP. Even so, diuretics have traditionally been a first-line choice for the treatment of HBP—even though they also tend to raise blood lipid levels.

5. *Calcium:* The idea is controversial, but a low-calcium intake may be related to HBP. Some studies have shown that replacing calcium in the diet helps normalize blood pressure. Calcium is an often overlooked nutrient. However, we only need to take it to the extent of our recommended daily allowances (see pages 110–111).

6. *Alcohol:* Regular alcohol consumption in excess has been shown to cause high blood pressure. One or two drinks per day probably does not do any harm. In excess of one or two per day there is a strong relationship between alcohol intake and high blood pressure. Some people with high blood pressure are very sensitive to alcohol, and even the two drinks a day may be too much.

    Having a few drinks every now and then is no problem, but if it is daily, then you should question why there is a need to drink. Maybe you have a problem?

7. *Stimulants:* Caffeine and nicotine are two commonly used stimulants. They have been related to the development and/or aggravation of HBP. Smoking at all times is bad; however, one or two cups of coffee or caffeinated beverage may not do you any harm. Consuming caffeine in excess of this not only will aggravate HBP but will also raise blood cholesterol levels.

8. *Stress:* Chronic stress may lead to repeated activation of the sympathetic nervous system and to the release of adrenaline, which will cause HBP. Stress is the most difficult factor to affect, as it is usually caused by some event beyond our control.

Correcting all the factors listed above should lower your blood pressure to optimal levels so that when you do get into a stressful situation, your pressure does not go up too high. You need a cushion to protect yourself because no matter how relaxed and laid back you are—when you are under stress, your blood pressure will rise.

Much of the processed food we eat is high in salt and low in calcium and potassium. We must begin to move away from prepackaged, processed foods and eat more fruits, vegetables, and fresh foods.

Eighty to eighty-five percent of people going through the HealthMark program will normalize their blood pressure and reduce or eliminate the need for blood pressure medication within 1 to 2 weeks, simply through the above changes. For these people, normal blood pressure will continue only if they adhere to the changes they have made in their lifestyles.

Two basic requirements are necessary: First, monitor daily your blood pressure with a blood pressure cuff. Digital blood pressure cuffs give reasonably accurate readings and are adequate. The regular type of blood pressure cuff with a built-in stethoscope that requires listening to the blood pressure is more accurate but more difficult to use. Purchase a unit of your choice; then go to your doctor's office, have the nurse show you how to use it, and check it against the office's blood pressure cuffs.

Second, medication should not be diminished or discontinued without the advice or supervision of your doctor. If your doctor is unwilling to change the medication and your blood pressure is normal, then go and find a doctor who is willing to work with you.

The bottom line is that you need a normal blood pressure at all times. How you get it there is of no real consequence. Obviously good nutrition and regular exercise are easy and effective ways to do this, and they have many other added benefits beyond the treatment of HBP. If medication is also required to control the blood pressure, then you need to take it.

The majority of people will be able to control their blood pressures with diet and exercise alone; in reality only a small percentage require medication.

DIABETES MELLITUS

There are 10 million diabetics in the United States, although many are unaware that they have diabetes. This disease is characterized by an elevation of the blood sugar. Such symptoms as excessive thirst, passing large amounts of urine, voracious appetite, and weight loss are related to the high blood sugar level. If the sugar level rises too high, diabetic coma can result.

The body handles sugar in a very specific way. Sugar (glucose) enters the bloodstream after being absorbed from the intestine and cannot readily get into the cells of the body without help. Sugar is the favorite fuel source of the body; it burns cleanly without any toxic breakdown products. Insulin, a hormone secreted by the pancreas (an organ in the abdomen which secretes other hormones and digestive juices as well), helps sugar get into the cells. When the blood sugar level rises, insulin is secreted in response. It works like a key opening a door to allow the sugar to pass from the blood into the cells.

When we don't have any insulin at all, sugar piles up in the blood and causes symptoms. We call this *juvenile diabetes*, or *type 1 diabetes*. This accounts for only 10 to 15 percent of all diabetes and usually occurs in children and young adults. In this disease the pancreas has stopped making insulin. People with juvenile diabetes will need to take insulin for the rest of their lives.

For most diabetics insulin is present in normal or even increased amounts. However, it is not working because these diabetics have become resistant to it. The key is present, but it no longer fits the lock and is unable to open the door to allow sugar into the cells. This is called *adult-onset* or *type 2 diabetes*, and it occurs mostly in adults. It is very easy to control, or even reverse, and accounts for 85 to 90 percent of all diabetes.

Diabetes is an extremely serious disease because of its complications. Prior to the discovery of insulin in the 1920s, diabetics died because of the high blood sugar levels and resulting coma. Today we have the "silver bullet" (insulin), but diabetics are suffering from the complications of the disease:

1. *Small-vessel disease:* The small arteries of the eye, kidney, and feet may be affected, resulting in kidney failure, leg ulcers, and gangrene as well as blindness (diabetes is a major cause of blindness in the United States).

2. *Large-vessel disease:* Diabetes accelerates the development of atherosclerosis, causing premature heart attacks, strokes, and peripheral vascular disease of the legs with gangrene.

3. *Nerve damage:* Damage to the peripheral nerves (peripheral neuropathy) of the hands and feet may cause tingling and eventual numbness. The spinal cord may also be involved.

The nerve damage and small-vessel disease may be avoided or controlled by close and tight regulation of the blood sugar levels. The hope here is that the closer we can approximate the normal blood sugar levels, the less these dreaded complications will occur.

The atherosclerotic complications should be preventable by controlling cholesterol levels and other cardiovascular risk factors. Traditional diabetic diets used in the Western world were high in proteins and fats and low in carbohydrates. Diabetics were advised to avoid carbohydrates because they are broken down into sugar that raises the blood sugar level. Recent evidence has shown that diabetics *can* handle most carbohydrates normally, especially the complex carbohydrate, and their intake should be encouraged. Unfortunately, when a high animal protein diet is eaten, excess fat and cholesterol cannot be avoided. These intensely high fat, high cholesterol diets may be partly responsible for the rampant atherosclerotic complications that diabetics suffer. In addition, there must be some contribution to the complications from the diabetes itself.

In India and Japan diets are much lower in fat and cholesterol than in the United States, and diabetics there have a much lower incidence of heart attack, stroke, and gangrene than do their counterparts in the United States. This phenomenon is probably related to the dietary difference.

As mentioned, in adult-onset diabetics, insulin is present in normal or increased amounts and is not working. Obesity, high fat diets, and lack of fiber and exercise have been known to contribute to this insulin resistance. Dr. James Anderson at the University of Kentucky showed that by simply changing the factors that caused insulin resistance, you can control the disease very easily. (Why these factors cause insulin resistance in some genetically predisposed individuals is unknown.)

We need to change the following factors in order to control adult-onset diabetes:

1. Lose weight (80 percent of adult-onset diabetics are too fat).

2. Eat a low fat diet.

3. Exercise.

4. Eat lots of fiber.

Through this approach of exercise; weight loss; and a low fat, high fiber, and high complex carbohydrate diet, Dr. Anderson was able to elicit some dramatic changes in adult-onset diabetes. Sixty percent of the diabetics were taken off insulin completely, and the remainder were able to lower their insulin requirements. Most patients taking oral medication can be taken off without any problem.

At HealthMark we have been able to duplicate these results and take adult-onset diabetics off insulin and oral medication in a short time. As with cardiovascular diseases, simply eating and exercising correctly may have a dramatic impact on the course of the disease. The genetic tendency is for the disease always to be there. However, it will only become symptomatic with the reinstitution of weight gain and poor eating and exercise habits.

By adapting the above principles and controlling other risk factors (HBP and smoking), the atherosclerotic vascular complications of diabetes may be greatly reduced, and the disease itself will be better controlled or eliminated.

CANCER

Many factors are involved in the development of cancer, e.g., occupational exposures, environmental hazards, viruses, and diet. All forms of cancer account for 20 percent (or 440,000) of all the deaths annually in the United States. It is estimated that 40 percent of cancers in men and 60 percent of cancers in women may be attributable to dietary factors. We will deal only with the diet-related factors in this section.

The evidence linking diet to the commoner types of cancer is so compelling that the National Academy of Sciences published a book entitled *Diet, Nutrition and Cancer* in 1982. The book lists the evidence linking high fat diets to the development of colon, breast, and prostate cancer. In addition, it lists cancers of the ovary, uterus, and pancreas as very likely candidates. Fortunately, the dietary recommendations it made are the same for heart attacks, high blood pressure, diabetes, obesity, and all the "Western diseases" already listed. We have, so to speak, a "one-diet cures-all."

Dietary Recommendations of the National Academy of Sciences

1. Reduce the total amount of fat consumed, both saturated and unsaturated.

2. Eat more fiber and foods containing vitamin C and carotene.

3. Reduce the consumption of salt-cured and smoked foods.

4. Remove the additives and contaminants in foods.

5. Stop smoking and reduce the consumption of alcohol.

There is a distinct geographical distribution of cancer in the world today. In the Western world there is an abundance of lung, colon, breast, and prostate cancers, whereas in the third world these cancers are relatively rare. Why? Not because of racial or genetic factors, because when we follow the migration of third-world people to the West, they rapidly develop the same types of cancer that are usually present there, sometimes within one generation.

The Japanese who migrated to the United States are an example of this. When their diets were "westernized," they switched from their traditionally low fat, low cholesterol, and high fiber diets to high fat, high cholesterol, and low fiber diets. As further evidence, in Japan the incidence of heart attacks and colon, breast, and prostate cancers has risen together with a rise in their intake of fat, i.e., a westernization of their eating habits.

Let us look at some of the most common types of cancers.

Lung Cancer

Lung cancer is the common form of cancer, accounting for 130,000 deaths annually. More than 80 percent of lung cancer cases are directly or indirectly (through passive smoking) related to smoking. If we all stopped smoking, lung cancer would fall from the number-one cancer death to an extremely rare form.

The death rate from lung cancer is rising faster in women than in men. In 1986 lung cancer surpassed breast cancer as the leading cancer death in women. Studies have shown that lung cancer death rates are leveling off in white men but are increasing in black men and white and black women. This is all related to smoking.

Smoking also is associated with cancers of the mouth, throat, larynx, and bladder. In addition, it causes emphysema and chronic bronchitis such that the ability of the lungs to oxygenate the blood is permanently impaired, eventually requiring continuous oxygen therapy. More people die from heart attacks induced by smoking than from cancers caused by smoking.

Smoking causes 360,000 deaths annually from the diseases listed above as well as heart attacks. It has been estimated that treatment of smoking-related diseases costs us $60 billion annually. The need to stop smoking is obvious.

Colon Cancer

There are 160,000 new cases diagnosed and 60,000 deaths annually from colon cancer. It is increasing in frequency each year. This is the second commonest cancer. If we stopped smoking, the decrease in incidence of lung cancer would make cancer of the colon number one. Two dietary factors set the stage for the development of colon cancer: fiber and fat.

Fiber

Lack of dietary fiber has been implicated in the development of many intestinal disorders. These include colon cancer, diverticulosis, appendicitis, and spastic colon.

The major function of fiber is to shorten the passage time of stool through the colon. Fiber is the nondigestible parts of food, such as cellulose, hemicellulose, and lignin. In the colon (or large intestine) the fiber forms bulk and draws water into it. This will cause you to have bulkier and looser bowel movements. The overall effect is to shorten the passage time of fecal contents through the intestine. Consequently, on a high fiber diet with a fast passage time, any irritants or cancer-causing agents present in the stool will not be able to spend much time irritating the colon and are whisked away. On a low fiber diet with resultant constipation, the harmful irritants are able to spend much time causing damage that will eventually set the stage for the development of polyps and cancer.

On a high fiber diet your stools should be loose and bulky, and you should have two to three stools per day. A firm, formed stool usually indicates constipation.

Fat

Ingestion of a high fat diet will cause two changes to occur. First, in response to the high fat intake, the liver increases the amount of bile that is secreted into the intestine. The function of bile is to emulsify the fat so that it can be absorbed. Second, the bacteria that normally live in the large intestine change from aerobic (oxygen-dependent), friendly bacteria to unfriendly anaerobic (oxygen-independent or resistant) bacteria.

When all this excess bile reaches the large intestine, it is attacked by the unfriendly bacteria, and two toxic bile salts are produced. These are cancer-promoting agents. If allowed to remain in the colon for a prolonged time, these agents will eventually set the stage for the development of polyps and cancer. The effect of a low fiber diet causing stasis and constipation obviously aggravates the situation by allowing the toxins to irritate the bowel for longer periods.

Interestingly enough, laboratory evidence has shown that any fat consumed in excess will cause these irritants to be produced. In fact, some studies have shown that polyunsaturated fats may be more harmful than saturated fats in the development of colon cancer. This is why the National Research Council recommended a total reduction of fat intake. It is obvious why a low fat, high fiber diet is recommended.

Traditional treatment for colon cancer is surgery and possibly radiation and chemotherapy. Although diet is all-important in the cause of this disease, it has only an adjunctive role in therapy. Patients with colon cancer should have a HealthMark type of nutrition program as part of their general health maintenance, but it should not be a mainstay of the therapy. This applies to all types of cancer.

Breast Cancer

About 100,000 new cases of breast cancer are diagnosed annually with 40,000 deaths each year. Breast cancer and lung cancer are the leading causes of cancer deaths in women. It is estimated that 1 in 11 women will develop breast cancer.

There is a significant relationship between fat intake and the development of breast cancer. For example, Japanese women traditionally have low incidence of breast cancer (one-sixth the rate of the United States). However, after emigration to the United States, the incidence of breast cancer in Japanese women equaled the incidence in Caucasian American women in the second generation.

This loss of protection against breast cancer correlated with the increase of dietary fat and may be most important in prepuberty.

A high fat diet causes obesity, and obese people are known to have higher estrogen levels. These higher levels lead to chronic overstimulation of breast and uterine tissue, possibly leading to the development of cancer in these organs. In addition, the higher estrogen levels in obese girls leads to early puberty, which in itself is a risk for breast cancer.

A strong family history of breast cancer in a mother or sister raises the risk, and thus added caution is needed. This is especially true if the breast cancer was premenopausal or in both breasts. The risk is less if the relative's cancer was only in one breast and occurred after menopause.

A woman's reproductive history also has a major role in determining her risk for breast cancer. The specific factors are:

1. Early onset of menstruation (before 12 years old)

2. Late menopause (after 50)

3. Not having children

4. Having a first child after 30

Other factors that may cause an increased risk are certain types of fibrocystic disease (not in women with typical fibrocystic disease with cysts, fibroadenomas, and fibrosis) and alcohol intake. Recent studies on alcohol intake showed that even moderate intake of alcohol was associated with increased risk. These studies are not conclusive. Women who have high risk should avoid alcohol or drink only occasionally until further evidence is available.

Protection against breast cancer should come primarily from a low fat diet. Unfortunately, once the disease is established, there is no evidence that diet plays a role in the therapy. Everyone with breast cancer should be on a low fat diet for general health reasons. The specific treatment for the cancer, however, should be with traditional means, such as surgery, chemotherapy, and radiation. Although diet may play a specific role in the development of breast cancer, it is used as an adjunct to usual therapy in the treatment of disease.

All your risks should be assessed, and if no major increased risk is present, the following guidelines for screening should be performed:

1. Monthly breast self-examinations

2. Yearly examinations by a physician

3. A screening mammogram between 35 and 40 years of age

4. Mammograms every 2 to 3 years after age 40

5. Mammograms annually after age 50

If your risk is elevated (especially from family history), then you should do all the above but begin mammograms earlier and do them more frequently, as per the advice of your physician. See Table 1-2 for a comparison of breast cancer risks.

Prostate Cancer

It is said that if all men in the Western world lived long enough, they would all develop cancer of the prostate. This is a rare cancer in the third world, but once again, when we look at emigration of Japanese men to the United States, the incidence of the disease in Japanese who emigrated rapidly equaled that of the Caucasian Americans, concomitant with the adoption of the typical American high fat diet.

A high fat diet will cause the production of more estrogen (female hormones), which in men will stimulate the production of more androgen (male hormone) receptors in the cells of the prostate. The resultant increased stimulation of the prostate by androgen may lead to prostate cancer.

Low fat diets are used as an adjunct to routine therapy for prostate cancer, such as surgery, radiation, and estrogen therapy. Estrogen has been implicated indirectly in the cause of prostate

Table 1-2   Comparison of Breast Cancer Risks

High Risk	Low Risk
Older than 50 years	Younger than 50 years
Cancer of the other breast	Both ovaries removed early in life
Family history of breast cancer	No family history of breast cancer
No pregnancies	One or more pregnancies
First child born after age 30	Full-term pregnancy before age 30
Onset of menstruation before age 12	Onset of menstruation after age 12
Menopause after age 50	Early menopause
Obesity	Slenderness
High fat diet	Low fat diet

cancer; however, it has also been shown to be effective in the treatment of it.

Other Cancers

There is also preliminary evidence to implicate high fat diets in the development of cancer of the ovary, uterus, and pancreas. The mechanisms for this relationship are unclear.

Other Factors That May Increase the Risk for Cancer

Emotions—Stress

Emotions are a difficult area to research, but there is growing interest in studying the relationships of stress and the development of cancer. Stress may lower your immune response and thus make you more susceptible to cancer.

A cancer-prone personality has also been characterized as a *Type C personality*. These people are characterized by:

Giving more than they receive in personal relationships

Repressing real anxieties and appearing to be strong and well-adjusted while they are actually emotionally insecure

Feeling an unusual amount of self-pity

Having an unhappy, stressful childhood

Being loners without an extensive support system

Worrying over small things

All these traits of trying to be someone you are not will over-stress your immune system. How life changes or emotional upsets affect cancer is unclear, but observations of some people who develop cancer show that they have recently undergone major life changes.

I developed my cancer 5 months after moving from Boston to Denver to begin a private practice. This was an enormous stress on my life and possibly was linked to my cancer. By the way, I exhibit some of the type C personality traits, and I am working hard to try to combat them.

Food Additives

Many food additives and preservatives have been linked to cancer. For a more detailed description, please refer to pages 124–128.

Barbecued or Smoked Foods

Large quantities of smoked fish and meats are bad because the smoking causes the release of polycyclic aromatic hydrocarbons, which are linked to stomach cancer.

In charcoal grilling and barbecuing, fat drips onto the hot coals, and the smoke coats the outside of the meat with hydrocarbons. Using low fat beef, chicken (without the skin), and fish should lessen this problem and enable us to barbecue more often. Once or twice a week is adequate.

The incidence of stomach cancer has been declining over the last 20 to 30 years, making us less concerned with this type of cancer; however, be cautious.

Coffee

Some studies have linked coffee in excess to cancer of the pancreas, and it does not seem to make a difference whether you drink regular or decaffeinated coffee. These studies are thought-provoking, but more research is necessary to reach definitive conclusions. However, these studies cannot be ignored. One or two cups of coffee per day is no problem.

Hormones

The use of diethylstilbestrol (DES) in the 1950s, 1960s, and 1970s to prevent miscarriage has given rise to the development of vaginal cancer in some of the female offspring of these women. Some of the children have developed vaginal cancer in their early twenties. If your mother took DES while she was pregnant with you, regular checkups are necessary for early detection. Please check with your gynecologist.

In addition, the women who actually took the DES may have an increased risk of breast cancer and need to have regular mammograms and do careful breast self-examinations.

Estrogen used to treat postmenopausal symptoms in women may increase the risk of cancer of the uterus. If a hysterectomy has been performed, however, estrogen therapy is no problem. Otherwise, estrogen should be taken in conjunction with progesterone. Regular Pap tests should be performed and careful attention paid to vaginal spotting (bleeding). If this bleeding develops, see your gynecologist as soon as possible.

Ultraviolet Light and Skin Cancer

Ultraviolet light and infrared waves cause damage to the cells of your skin and can lead to cancer. Darkly pigmented people are protected by the melanin (pigment) in their skin, whereas lightly pigmented people are at risk. Prolonged, excessive use of infrared tanning booths may also damage skin and increase risk for skin cancer.

The exposure to sunlight is cumulative. The more you are exposed, the greater your risk of developing skin cancer. Severe sunburns in children are related to the later development of skin cancer.

Skin cancers may be the superficial basal cell cancers easily treated with surgery or "burning off." Squamous cell cancers are more serious because they can spread, although they are usually superficial and localized. Melanoma is the dangerous skin cancer and develops in pigmented skin moles. Occasionally it can spread and be fatal. Beware of any mole that changes pigmentation or begins to bleed and ulcerate and any skin lesion that fails to heal or is chronic. Have them checked out by a dermatologist.

Don't worship the sun. A suntan may look good, but it ages your skin (dries it out and wrinkles it) and predisposes you to skin cancer. Use sunscreens containing *para*-aminobenzoic acid (PABA) with a sun protection factor (SPF) of 15 or more. They are available in SPF 25 and 29. The higher the number, the better the sunscreen will block the sun. Use the sunscreens that don't wash off with water and sweat.

Radiation

Radiation has strongly been associated with cancer, particularly in people with excessive exposure, such as atomic blasts. Low levels of chronic exposure to radiation will also increase the cancer risk.

X-ray treatment (radiation) was used to treat tonsillitis and acne in the 1940s and 1950s. The people who received radiation around the face and neck are at higher risk for developing thyroid nodules and thyroid cancer. If you had this type of radiation, you should have your thyroid checked frequently.

Be aware of unnecessary x-rays, and keep an eye on your doctor and dentist in ordering them. The American Cancer Society no longer recommends routine chest x-rays, and x-rays should only be done for diagnostic purposes, not for screening.

Environmental Pollutants

Within our homes and workplaces we should make every effort to avoid exposure to agents that may cause cancer. Chemical wastes are continuously being disposed of in the water and air.

Houses that are too well insulated keep heat in but may also keep harmful fumes and chemicals in the air. Always keep your house well ventilated, especially when working with chemicals. The following chemicals and substances are known cancer-causing agents:

Arsenic: Used in pesticides, paints, and wood preservatives. It is also a by-product of smelting copper and lead.

Asbestos: Used in fireproofing, insulation, wallboards, brake linings, caulking, roofing, and flooring.

Benzene: Used in gasoline, adhesives, pesticides, inks, and paints.

Ethylene dibromide (EDB): Found in pesticides and leaded gasoline.

Formaldehyde: Used in plastics, building materials, foam insulation, embalming fluid, soil fumigants, room deodorants, and cosmetics. It is used to decaffeinate most coffee unless stated to be Swiss water processed (see Chapter 3).

Hair dye: 4-methoxy-*M* phenylenediamine (4MMPD).

Nickel: Used in alloy form, in shipbuilding and aerospace technology.

Polychlorinated biphenyl: Used in pesticides and electric industry; banned but still in use.

Vinyl chloride: A gaseous material used in plastics and floor tile. Now banned from plastic wrap and bottles.

Considering that approximately 90 percent of cancers are environmental in origin from smoking, nutrition, and environmental hazards, we should be a little more cautious and possibly prevent cancer from becoming our leading cause of death.

We can prevent many more cancers from developing than we can cure with the therapy we have available.

Smoking

Smoking is one of the most difficult risk factors to control. It has tremendous health implications and is the cause of a huge amount of both suffering and enjoyment. Therein lies the problem. We use smoking for enjoyment. It is a crutch, a pacifier, a stimulant, and nicotine is one of the most addictive substances available.

According to surveys, over two-thirds of smokers in the United States would like to quit. Most of the adults who smoke are aware of the health risks of smoking and yet are unable to give it up. Smoking kills approximately 360,000 people in this country annually, and about $60 billion is spent to treat smoking-related diseases.

What Are the Health Risks of Smoking?

1. *Emphysema and chronic bronchitis:* These diseases occur after years of smoking damage. The lung tissue literally dissolves so that oxygen cannot be passed into the blood. This is not reversible, but the damage is not progressive when you stop smoking. The damage is extremely debilitating and, if far enough advanced, will cause the need for continuous oxygen therapy and the lack of capacity for any exertion.

2. *Heart disease:* It is said that for every three people who smoke, only one gets lung cancer (this is the good news), and the other two will have heart attacks (this is the bad news). In fact, more people die each year from smoking-induced heart attacks than from lung cancer.

3. *Lung cancer:* The majority of lung cancers are caused by smoking, either active or passive. If smoking were stopped completely, lung cancer would become extremely rare instead of the leading cause of death by cancer—130,000 deaths annually.

4. *Other cancers:* Cancers of the mouth, throat, larynx (vocal cords), and bladder are related to smoking.

5. *Allergies:* Allergies are commonly associated with smoking, as are recurrent bronchial and upper respiratory infections.

The good news is that if you stop smoking, the risk for heart attack and lung cancer is reduced. Heart attack risk rates fall off dramatically after you quit smoking, and risk is halved in 1 year; however, it takes 5 to 10 years for the risk of lung cancer or heart attack to fall to that of someone who has never smoked.

It is not easy to stop smoking; it might be one of the hardest things you will ever do. Some people find it easy to quit, but they are the exception rather than the rule. It is the fear of quitting that prevents most people from doing it.

The first step is to make up your mind that you have to do it. No stop-smoking program will work unless you want it to work. *Make up your mind to do it.*

The next step is to understand what you will go through. You will experience *withdrawal,* and there are two phases.

Phase 1: The physical withdrawal from nicotine, a stimulant. You may get a lot of nonspecific symptoms such as headaches, light-headedness, inability to concentrate, sleepiness, and lethargy. Being a stimulant, nicotine also depresses the appetite and increases the metabolism. The absence of nicotine will slow the metabolism and account for some of the weight gain experienced with quitting smoking.

Phase 2: The psychological withdrawal. This withdrawal will persist for years after quitting. It is the craving and associations that we tend to have with cigarettes, such as after a meal and while having a drink. A lot of time is required to completely get over this phase. It took me 3 to 4 years to detest cigarette smoke.

Understanding these phases will help you stop. You can overcome many of the nicotine withdrawal symptoms with the use of Nicorette gum. The gum contains nicotine and can be used under the guidance of your physician in decreasing doses over a 2-week period. It must be prescribed by a physician.

Quitting smoking is a very negative event. You are giving up something you like and depend upon, and usually it is replaced with food craving, the need to have something in your mouth. This can be overcome by chewing gum or by biting on plastic-tipped cigars without lighting them. Excess food intake combined with a slower metabolism leads to weight gain. Depression results from not having the nicotine (the stimulant) and from the weight gain. It can be overcome by exercising and eating well.

In the HealthMark program we encourage people to give up smoking before they begin the program, and we see excellent results. The negative (withdrawal and depression) is replaced with something positive (exercising and eating well). You are doing something positive (exercising and eating well) to reinforce the lifestyle change, and you won't gain weight. All the good feelings that you experience with the HealthMark program far outweigh the negative symptoms of giving up smoking.

I can tell you that all the stop-smoking programs, hypnosis, and acupuncture or acupressure will work only if you want them to. Use whatever help you need to give up smoking—just give it up. Some people need two or three attempts before they are successful. I needed two.

OSTEOPOROSIS

Loss of calcium from bones will cause them to become thinned and to fracture easily. Fractures of the hip are the most devastating consequence of osteoporosis. The fractured head of the femur, the thigh bone (so-called hip fracture), will not heal and requires an artificial hip. This usually occurs at an advanced age and therefore may have disastrous consequences. Estimates are that 40,000 to 50,000 people die each year within 3 to 6 months of sustaining the hip fracture. In addition, one-third of these patients will require long-term care facilities and never regain their former social status or physical function. It has been estimated that it costs us more than $6 billion per year to treat and care for patients with osteoporosis-related fractures.

Approximately 1.2 million fractures per year occur as a result of osteoporosis: 538,000 fractures in the spine, 227,000 in the hip, and 172,000 in the wrist. It has been estimated that for those who live to the age of 90, one in three women and one in six men will have had a hip fracture.

Women get osteoporosis twice as often as men. The loss of calcium from the bone begins after the age of 35. Many factors contribute to calcium loss from the bone, thus causing osteoporosis:

1. *Race:* White or Oriental females are most at risk. The disease is rare in blacks.

2. *Family history:* A history of the disease is present in 90 percent of all cases.

3. *Early menopause:* Oophorectomy (removal of the ovaries) is just as often a factor.

4. *Low calcium intake:* This is by far the most important nutritional factor, as people on high calcium diets will have many fewer hip fractures than people on low calcium diets. Calcium replacements do not appear to help prevent further bone loss, and the role of calcium is more in prevention.

    To attain daily calcium balance, so that the net effect of calcium intake versus calcium loss is positive, you need the following amounts of calcium:

Men: 800 mg/day

Women: premenopausal, 1000 mg/day

Women: postmenopausal, 1500 mg/day

Dietary calcium is one of the most overlooked nutrients. The average American woman consumes less calcium than the average American male. The average intake for postmenopausal women is 500 mg per day, which is 1000 mg less than should be consumed to maintain calcium balance. See Chapter 4 for calcium sources in food.

5. *High protein intake:* Even in the presence of an adequate calcium intake, a high protein intake will cause calcium loss from bone. The traditional U.S. diet is very high in protein and may contribute significantly to the development of osteoporosis, and therefore we need to deemphasize the importance of protein as a nutrient. (See Chapter 3.)

6. *High caffeine intake:* Small amounts of caffeine probably are not harmful.

7. *High alcohol intake:* This is an important risk factor in men as well as young, premenopausal women, particularly if there is chronic alcohol abuse.

8. *Sedentary lifestyle:* Inactivity leads to calcium loss from the bones; exercise will help prevent this loss.

9. *Cigarette smoking:* The reason for this association is not yet clear.

10. *Pregnancy and the use of oral contraceptives:* These may increase bone mass in the fertile phase of life and may protect against the development of significant bone loss. This is due to the positive effect of estrogen.

11. *Other factors:* These include whether one takes cortisone or has type 1 diabetes or an overactive thyroid gland.

The therapy of osteoporosis obviously is in prevention. Adequate amounts of calcium need to be taken either by diet or calcium supplementation. Not all calcium supplements, however, are absorbed effectively. To test the absorbability of your calcium supplement, place a tablet of it in any kind of vinegar. About 75 percent of the tablet should disintegrate within 30 minutes, indicating that it will be broken down by the acid in your stomach and absorbed. Among the best sources of absorbable calcium are Oscal, Caltrate, Tums, Biocal, oyster shell calcium (from Fields of Nature, Giant Foods, and Nature Made), and HiCal (from Safeway). Taking calcium in large quantities, above the recommended allowances, has not been shown to prevent or delay the onset of osteoporosis. Therefore, we need to get our recommended daily allowance of calcium, and we must also limit the factors that promote calcium loss, such as high intakes of protein, caffeine, nicotine, and alcohol. In addition, regular weight-bearing aerobic exercise must be performed. Once menopause sets in, the question of estrogen replacement needs to be addressed. If replacement of estrogen is begun soon after menopause starts, the evidence shows that calcium loss can be prevented. However, if replacement is begun more than 5 years after menopause has set in, the calcium loss may not be preventable.

The question of estrogen replacement is still being debated. The only complication is the increased risk for the development of cancer of the uterus. The general consensus today is that if you have had a hysterectomy, the risk is obviously not there and estrogen replacement should be given. If you have not had a hysterectomy, then the estrogen should be given with progesterone and regular Pap tests should be performed to detect possible abnormalities. Obviously, if uterine bleeding or spotting occurs, it should be investigated immediately.

The sad fact is that once the calcium is gone from the bones, it is very difficult to replenish.

THE PERIODIC MEDICAL EVALUATION

Feeling good is unfortunately not enough, because you can be ill and not know it. You may also have seriously elevated risk factors, such as blood pressure and cholesterol levels, and unknowingly be a walking time bomb.

Most walking time bombs will eventually admit that they don't feel quite right, but they are usually deniers. Once they go through a successful HealthMark lifestyle change, they will tell you how great they feel now and that they did not know how poorly they actually felt before the change.

Should We Have Periodic Medical Examinations?

The answer is definitely yes. We need to go through periodic examinations to provide the necessary disease and risk factor detection. Many people have medical evaluations that may be a waste of time. No medical problems are found, but risks that develop into medical problems are ignored or glossed over. You keep going back for routine evaluations until something is found. This is a very negative approach.

Obviously, the patient is not at fault. He or she wants to make sure that everything is okay. It is the medical examiner who is at fault. Not enough time is spent evaluating risk and teaching risk factor modification. In the traditional annual physical, the patient is usually told "everything is fine; come back next year." It's great that nothing is found, but beyond this it is useless.

You want to be sure of covering two separate areas when you go for the periodic physical examination.

1. *Disease detection:* You need to go often enough to make sure that all the necessary disease detection procedures are performed. You also want to detect problems early so they can be treated early and cured.

2. *Risk detection and education:* The risk factors for our leading causes of death, such as cardiovascular disease, cancer, high blood pressure, and diabetes, should be evaluated. Then adequate education should be given to show you how to reverse them.

Don't wait for something to happen before you decide to make some change—it may be too late then.

A complete physical exam should be done at regular intervals:

Under the age of 30, every 3 to 5 years

From 30 to 40 years of age, every 2 to 3 years

Above 40 years of age, every 1 to 2 years

Above 50 years of age, annually

If you have risk factors, the frequency of periodic physicals should be increased until these factors are controlled or normalized.

What Should Be Done in Your Periodic Physical?

1. A complete history and physical exam by an internist or family practice physician.

2. Blood testing to include a complete chemistry survey (sugar, liver function, kidney function, electrolytes, and thyroid function), lipid profile (cholesterol, triglycerides, HDL, LDL, and cholesterol-HDL ratio), and blood counts.

3. Urinalysis.

4. Rectal examination after the age of 40 or sooner if symptoms are present (e.g., hemorrhoids).

5. Three stool tests for hidden blood after the age of 35.

6. Routine pelvic examination and Pap test, annually.

7. Hearing tests.

8. Vision screening.

9. Glaucoma screening.

10. Pulmonary (lung) function test.

11. Chest x-ray should never be done as routine, except for smokers. The American Cancer Society no longer recommends routine chest x-rays because of the unnecessary radiation.

12. Treadmill stress test—after the age of 35 and earlier if any cardiac risk factors are present.

13. Flexible sigmoidoscopy, which uses a flexible tube passed into the rectum to check for hemorrhoids, polyps, or cancer. This should be done only if there is blood in the stool and routinely every 2 to 3 years after the age of 50.

14. Height, weight, and body fat measurements.

15. Mammograms, which should be routinely done between 35 and 40 and then every 2 to 3 years after the age of 40 and annually after the age of 50. If there is high risk (positive family history), then yearly from a younger age.

16. Resting electrocardiograms—as routine screening tests they don't tell very much; as diagnostic tests they are good, e.g., for chest pain.

What Tests Can We Do on Our Own?

1. Have your cholesterol and other lipids checked every 2 to 3 months at a doctor's office or medical center until they are normalized, and then once a year.

2. Do stool tests for hidden blood annually after the age of 35. (Stool-testing kits are available at pharmacies.)

3. Check blood pressure periodically at supermarkets, health fairs, and so on. If you have high blood pressure, buy a blood pressure cuff and monitor it daily at home and keep a record to show your physician.

4. Do regular monthly breast self-examinations.

5. Do regular monthly testicular self-examinations.

6. Routinely check your skin for moles that are changing color or bleeding or new lesions that won't heal.

It is our responsibility to have periodic examinations and to make sure we are getting the necessary tests and not unnecessary tests. Unfortunately, some institutions still do unnecessary x-ray procedures, such as routine barium enemas and upper gastrointestinal (GI) examinations (bowel x-rays) as well as chest x-rays. These are good diagnostic tests but give too much radiation and too little yield (in picking up early disease) to be recommended as screening tests.

You need to assume responsibility for taking care of yourself and for finding the best medical help. Follow-up is also your responsibility to make sure that the problems and risks identified are attended to and normalized.

TWO

Danger: Cholesterol Ahead

Let us examine the specific relationship between food and disease. As mentioned, the food we eat and the leading causes of death are significantly related.

HOW DOES ATHEROSCLEROSIS BEGIN?

Atherosclerosis begins when cholesterol is deposited in the walls of arteries. Eventually, these deposits can cause blockage and obstruct blood flow. The symptoms that develop from the blocked artery depend on the site of the blockage. A blockage in the head or neck will result in a stroke; in the coronary arteries, a heart attack results; in the legs, gangrene may result, and aneurysms (a ballooning of the arteries) may form that can rupture with severe or fatal consequences. Atherosclerosis via heart attacks and strokes (cardiovascular diseases) is the leading cause of death in the United States today.

Initially cholesterol builds up in the inner lining of the arteries. These deposits are called fatty streaks, and we can actually see yellow streaks going up and down an artery. As it progresses, a plaque begins to form and bulges into the lumen (opening) of the artery. In the early stages it is soft and mushy; later, fibrous (scar) tissue and calcium are laid down and the plaque becomes hardened.

Symptoms will not develop until there is a 70 percent or more blockage. This indicates that the disease will progress silently for many years; by the time you develop symptoms, there is a major problem. Fortunately, we are able to control or even reverse this plaque.

Autopsy studies done on children who have died from accidental causes have shown that fatty streaks begin to develop after the age of 3. Autopsy studies done on the U.S. soldiers killed in Korea showed that 22-year-old men already had significant blockages in their coronary arteries, from fatty streaks to complete occlusions. Coronary artery disease may begin very early in life and will progress depending on the severity and number of risk factors present.

THE RISK FACTORS

The major risk factors are cholesterol, blood pressure, smoking, and diabetes. The minor factors are age, sex, obesity, triglycerides, personality type, lack of exercise, and family history.

> *Cholesterol*: Atherosclerosis begins and ends with cholesterol as the main player. Elevated levels of blood cholesterol or abnormalities in other blood lipids (see page 47) will cause cholesterol to be deposited in the walls of arteries. Risk for heart attack begins to rise when the blood cholesterol level reaches 182 milligrams per deciliter of blood (mg/dl). We can assume that at this level we are already depositing cholesterol in the arterial wall. As the level rises above 182 mg/dl, the rate increases at which this deposit occurs. Children born with cholesterol levels over 500 mg/dl (from genetic disorders) may have heart attacks before they become teenagers.

> *High blood pressure*: As the blood pressure rises above 140/90 (the upper limits of normal), the pressure generated in the arteries damages their inner lining (mechanical trauma) and allows cholesterol to pass from the blood into the artery wall more rapidly; i.e., it accelerates cholesterol deposit.

Smoking: Smoking damages the artery in two ways: First, the carbon monoxide inhaled (smoke) will damage the inner lining of the artery and allow cholesterol to pass into the wall at an accelerated rate. Second, the nicotine then causes the artery to constrict, which further narrows it, and this will cause premature heart attacks and strokes. Between 1965 and 1980, 3 million people in their early fifties or younger died in the United States from heart attacks and strokes prematurely induced by smoking.

Diabetes: This disease generally accelerates cholesterol deposits in the arteries. Diabetics have a much higher rate of heart attack and stroke than nondiabetics. The exact reason for this is unknown; however, it may result from the diabetes itself and/or the high fat, high cholesterol diets that diabetics traditionally have eaten under the guise of high protein.

Age: As we get older our cholesterol levels and blood pressure tend to rise, and so we get heart attacks and strokes. In cultures where people eat low fat, low cholesterol, and high fiber diets and are physically active (e.g., the Tarahumara Indians in central Mexico), their blood pressures and cholesterol levels remain normal throughout life, and the people don't get heart attacks and strokes.

Sex: Women are protected from heart attacks until menopause by estrogen, which elevates the level of protective, or good, high-density lipoprotein (HDL) cholesterol (described later). After menopause estrogen levels decrease, and the incidence of heart attacks soon catches up to that of men. By the age of 60 the incidence is equal to men, partly because some of the men have already died from heart attacks and also from the decrease that occurs in HDL in women.

Triglycerides: Triglyceride counts are the actual measurements of fat levels in the blood. An elevation of them will place you at increased risk. When elevated triglycerides are found in conjunction with a low HDL (or good cholesterol level), as they often are, the risk for heart attack and stroke may be significant.

Obesity: The link with obesity may be due to the associated risks that accompany it, e.g., elevated cholesterol levels and high blood pressure.

Lack of exercise: Recent evidence suggests that we need to exercise more than we thought. It appears that 18 to 20 miles of fast walking or jogging per week is needed for cardiovascular protection. This translates into about 40 to 45 minutes of exercise at least four to five times a week.

Family history: Some families have a strong history of heart attack at a young age. This usually indicates a genetic disorder in which some or all members of the family have an inability to excrete cholesterol. In other families the risk is less clearly defined.

Personality type: People with type A personalities (see Chapter 7) may be at increased risk because of this trait.

Each risk adds to the development of atherosclerosis and heart attack. If we begin to combine these risks, then we compound the overall risk. In some people the number and combination of risks is so great that we call them "walking time bombs." The tragedy is that almost all the risk factors are reversible and preventable.

Because cholesterol and fat are so important in the development of atherosclerosis, we should look at them in more detail.

IS THERE AN IDEAL CHOLESTEROL LEVEL?

The lowest blood cholesterol level we ever have is at birth: 79 to 90 mg/dl. Soon after birth the level begins to elevate. The increase is determined by the amount of fat and cholesterol you eat and the ability of your body to excrete cholesterol, and this ability is genetically determined. Each one of us excretes cholesterol at a different rate, and this explains why people can eat the same amounts of cholesterol and yet have different blood cholesterol levels.

The Tarahumara Indians in central Mexico eat very low fat, low cholesterol, and high fiber diets. The average blood cholesterol levels in their children is 116 mg/dl, and in the adults the average is 125 mg/dl. The average levels for U.S. children and adults are 180 mg/dl and 215 mg/dl, respectively. The Tarahumara do not get heart attacks. The Japanese traditionally had low levels of cholesterol, less than 160 mg/dl. Unfortunately, the level has been rising with a concomitant rise in the incidence of heart attacks. This has occurred because of the westernization of their diet with increased fat and cholesterol consumption. A similar phenomenon occurred in the Japanese who emigrated to the United States. The average blood cholesterol in Japan has risen to 190 mg/dl, and in the Japanese living in the United States, it is the same as the national average.

Data from a variety of different population studies are clear-cut. Those with the highest blood cholesterol levels have the highest incidence of heart attack, and this, in turn, correlates with the highest intake of saturated fat and cholesterol. Conversely, the lowest incidence of heart attacks is seen in the people with the lowest blood cholesterol levels and the lowest fat and cholesterol intakes, e.g., the Japanese, the Bantu in South Africa, and the Tarahumara Indians. When these people westernize their diets by adding more saturated fat and cholesterol, their blood cholesterol levels rise along with an increased rate of heart attacks.

The average blood cholesterol in the United States is 215 mg/dl. This is obtained from measuring levels in many people and determining the "normal" range. The normal range goes from 150 to 300 mg/dl. This reflects the range of cholesterol in the general population and does not mean it is ideal. We are eating an extremely high fat, high cholesterol diet, and as the blood levels are affected by our diet, this range does not reflect the truly normal values but rather our poor eating habits. When you are told by your medical adviser that "your cholesterol is normal; don't worry about it," my advice to you is to worry about it. This usually means that your cholesterol falls in the so-called normal range.

We know from population studies that 50 percent of all heart attacks occur at a blood cholesterol level between 150 and 245 mg/dl and the other 50 percent occur above 245 mg/dl. Thus we can see that 100 percent of heart attacks occur in the so-called normal range. You do not get cholesterol deposits in the arteries and have subsequent heart attacks without an elevated blood cholesterol level; therefore, these ranges of normal must be wrong. If you are in this range, you may be right on track for having a heart attack.

Heart attacks are not usually seen in any of the studies at a blood cholesterol level below 150 mg/dl. In fact we already begin to see the risk for heart attack rise at a level of 182 mg/dl. The higher your cholesterol level rises, the greater the risk; e.g., at a level of 220 mg/dl it is twice that of normal. At 250 mg/dl it is 3 times, and at 300 mg/dl it is 4 times that of normal. If you are a 45-year-old man or woman, your risk may be elevated 2, 3, 4, or more times (depending on concomitant risks) for getting a heart attack in 5 to 8 years; 50 percent of these events may be fatal. Your odds may be better at Russian roulette.

In October 1987 the National Institutes of Health issued the new cholesterol guidelines shown in Table 2-1. The ideal level is 200 mg/dl or less. *The HealthMark goal is 160 mg/dl or less.*

An easy rule of thumb is to say that the blood cholesterol should be 100 plus your age, and you stop counting at 60. There is some variability in this based on what the HDL level (good cholesterol) and cholesterol-HDL ratio are.

Table 2-1   New Cholesterol Guidelines

Total Cholesterol (mg/dl)	LDL Cholesterol (mg/dl)	Comment
< 200	< 130	Ideal
200–239	130–159	Borderline to high risk
> 240	> 160	High risk

GOOD AND BAD CHOLESTEROL

The total cholesterol level is made up of three fractions, one measuring good cholesterol and two bad. These fractions are called *lipoproteins*. Lipoprotein is a combination of the words *lipid* and *protein*. *Lipid* is the medical term for fat and cholesterol, and *protein* is the substance that carries lipid from place to place in the body. This can be likened to the dairy truck that comes to your house once or twice a week. The truck is like the protein, and in the back of the truck is all the fat and cholesterol.

The three lipoproteins are:

High-density lipoprotein (HDL), which is good

Low-density lipoprotein (LDL), which is bad

Very low density lipoprotein (VLDL), which is one-fifth of the triglyceride level (blood fats) and is bad

Thus the total cholesterol is HDL plus LDL plus one-fifth of triglyceride level or VLDL.

HDL (Good Cholesterol)

HDL is called "good" cholesterol because it reflects the cholesterol being taken out of your body (scavenger cholesterol). The HDL helps transport excess cholesterol from the storage sites, including the arteries, to the liver, where some of it is incorporated into bile and excreted into the intestine. Bile is the pigment that makes your stool brown. Most of the bile is reabsorbed from the intestine, and only a small amount is lost in the stool.

When the HDL levels are high, you are protected from heart attack, and thus the higher the level, the better. You can never have a high enough HDL. When the HDLs are low, the risk of heart attack is elevated.

HDLs are not influenced by diet. Nice, high HDLs are normally present if you choose good parents (i.e., you have good genes)

or if you are a woman. The only ways you can realistically raise your HDLs are to exercise, lose weight, and stop smoking; i.e., lack of exercise, obesity, and smoking depress HDL levels and therefore increase risk for heart disease.

Estrogen keeps the level of HDL up. As mentioned, after menopause women's estrogen and HDL levels decline, and the incidence of heart attacks increases in women to equal that of men. Progesterone lowers HDL as does testosterone. When athletes take anabolic steroids (testosterone), HDL levels decrease drastically. An athlete with very low levels of HDL is probably on steroids.

There are five types of HDL—HDL-1 through HDL-5. HDL-2 is the protective type; HDL-3 is apparently the type that is elevated by alcohol consumption and may not be protective. Thus the theory of two drinks a day may not hold much water. The alcohol effect on HDL is controversial, and no one should recommend two drinks a day to raise your HDL because of the inherent dangers of chronic alcohol ingestion (possible addiction and liver damage). It is better to raise your HDL with exercise, weight loss, and stopping smoking.

Causes of Reduced HDL

Smoking	Progesterone
Obesity	Testosterone
Lack of exercise	Elevated blood triglycerides (fats)
Blood pressure medication	Elevated blood cholesterol
Androgenic (anabolic) steroids	Bad genes

Normal Levels for HDL

The higher the level of HDL, the better—you can never have enough. Men should have a level of 45 mg/dl or greater. The level for women should be 55 mg/dl or greater (it is higher because of estrogen).

LDL (Bad Cholesterol)

Low-density lipoprotein (LDL) is called "bad" cholesterol because it is the cholesterol being deposited in the arterial wall, or artery-plugging cholesterol. The higher the LDL level, the greater the risk for developing heart attacks. We want this level as low as possible.

Eating cholesterol and saturated fats will raise the LDL level; i.e., it is influenced by diet. In addition, some people have genetic disorders (inherited) and are unable to excrete LDL at the normal rate and will have very high levels of LDL and total cholesterol.

Factors that Raise LDL Levels

Diet: Eating saturated fat and cholesterol
Bad genes: Inability to get rid of (excrete) LDL

The ideal values for LDL are 110 mg/dl or less. Acceptable levels are 130 mg/dl or less.

VLDL (Bad Cholesterol)

Very low density lipoprotein (VLDL) carries mostly triglycerides (fats) and a small amount of bad cholesterol. One-fifth of the triglyceride measurement contributes to the total cholesterol level. High levels of VLDL are seen in people with high triglycerides, and this is usually associated with a low HDL, causing a significant risk for heart attack. VLDL or triglycerides are also affected by diet.

Factors that Raise VLDL

Alcohol

Sugar

Excess calories

Obesity

Lack of exercise

The ideal values for VLDL are 25 mg/dl or less. Acceptable levels are less than 150 mg/dl.

Triglycerides

Triglycerides are the actual measurement of fat in the blood. They are the major component of the VLDL and are affected by the same factors. You need to fast 10 to 12 hours before measuring triglycerides.

Factors that Raise Triglycerides

Alcohol

Sugar

Excess calories

Obesity

Lack of exercise

Ideal values for triglycerides are less than 110 mg/dl. Acceptable level are less than 150 mg/dl.

THE ALL-IMPORTANT CHOLESTEROL/HDL RATIO

The cholesterol-HDL ratio is extremely important. It should be 3.5 or less.

Recent evidence suggests that this ratio really determines risk for heart attack and whether we are going to be able to stop and then reverse cholesterol buildup.

Most heart attacks occur when the ratio is between 5 and 6. An ideal level is below 3.5.

The variability in the total cholesterol is based on this ratio and more specifically the HDL level. Table 2-2 shows the cholesterol-HDL ratio and attendant risk level for four people.

Arnold: At first glance Arnold's cholesterol appears a little elevated; however, he has a high HDL level and a low ratio. Thus the cardiac risk is low, and 210 mg is a "normal" cholesterol for him.

Betty: Betty has a lower HDL, and the ratio is 5.2. Therefore, her risk is elevated.

Charlie: Charlie's cholesterol is low and appears to be at a safe level, but watch out. The HDLs are also low, and thus his ratio is elevated, and his risk is high. This pattern is usually seen with an elevated triglyceride level.

Donna: Donna's cholesterol is extremely high, and yet her HDLs are very high with a normal ratio. Don't be fooled. This pattern is sometimes seen in women, and in my experience the risk is elevated because the LDL has become severely elevated, negating the effect of the high HDL.

The ratio is probably only significant at the low and middle range of total cholesterol, but not at the very high end or when the LDL is above 130 mg/dl. We don't normally see heart attacks in people with total cholesterol levels below 150 mg/dl; however, there are two exceptions: people with very low HDLs (see above) and people who abuse cocaine. Cocaine can induce heart attacks at any time by causing severe spasm of the coronary arteries, independent of the cholesterol level or whether cholesterol deposits are present in the arteries. This spasm causes a complete blockage of the artery with a resultant heart attack.

All these risk factors need to be evaluated individually and collectively to adequately assess the risk for developing heart attacks.

Table 2-2   Ratio of Cholesterol to High-Density Lipoproteins (HDL)

	Total Cholesterol (mg/dl)	HDL (mg/dl)	Ratio of Cholesterol to HDL	Risk
Arnold	210	70	3.0	Low
Betty	210	40	5.2	High
Charlie	150	30	5.0	High
Donna	360	120	3.0	High

Knowing your cholesterol level is not enough. You need to know all your lipoprotein levels as well.

The average person headed for a heart attack or stroke usually has total cholesterol levels above 200 mg, low HDLs, and elevated cholesterol-HDL ratios. If you wait for chest pains to develop before deciding to make some changes in your lifestyle, you may be too late.

WHAT CAUSES THE BLOOD CHOLESTEROL LEVEL TO RISE?

There are two main reasons for blood cholesterol levels to rise: (1) diet and (2) genetics.

Dietary Factors

The consumption of saturated fat and cholesterol will predictably raise the blood cholesterol levels. Cholesterol is found only in animal foods. Saturated fat (fat that is solid at room temperature) is also found mostly in animal foods, also in coconut oil, palm oil, cocoa butter, and hydrogenated fats. In fact, this type of fat may raise your blood cholesterol more efficiently than dietary cholesterol itself. Cholesterol is only found in red meats, poultry, fish (all animal flesh), and dairy products. All these foods, with the exception of fish, also contain saturated fats, and thus when eaten will cause the "double whammy." Both saturated fat and cholesterol will independently raise your blood cholesterol levels, and together they do a big job. Fish contains polyunsaturated fat, which actually lowers cholesterol levels.

Genetic Factors

It is not that we manufacture too much cholesterol; rather, we excrete too little of it, causing our blood cholesterol levels to rise.

Everyone excretes cholesterol at a different rate. So if we take 100 people who all have elevated cholesterol levels and place them on the same cholesterol-lowering diet, they will all lower their cholesterol levels at different rates and to different levels. Conversely, if they all eat a very high fat and high cholesterol diet, their cholesterol levels will all rise at different rates to different heights.

The rate at which your cholesterol level rises or falls depends on how you get rid of it, and this is genetically determined. Most people can lower their cholesterol levels simply by lowering their saturated fat and cholesterol intake. However, a small percentage of people (10 to 15 percent) have difficulty lowering their cholesterol levels because of their genetic background. They will require medication in addition to the diet to optimally lower their cholesterol and lipid levels. These people will usually have a strong family history of heart attack and stroke.

A high level of LDL cholesterol will also inhibit cholesterol excretion. As the level lowers we become more efficient at excreting cholesterol.

GOOD AND BAD FAT

Some fat is good for you. Fat is designated good or bad by its effect on blood cholesterol levels; i.e., good fats lower it and bad fats raise it. The bad fats are saturated (animal or solid fat), and the good fats are unsaturated. These unsaturated fats are further divided into polyunsaturated fats derived from vegetable and fish oils and monounsaturated fats derived from nuts, olives, and avocados.

Why don't we keep our diet the same and add large amounts of these good fats to counter the effects of all the saturated fat and cholesterol we eat? Unfortunately, it is not that simple. Too much of any fat (in particularly polyunsaturated fat) can be harmful by causing obesity, gallstones, and possibly colon cancer.

The best guide is to eliminate as much saturated fat as possible and to eat only small quantities of unsaturated fats. Eskimos and certain Mediterranean people, who eat lots of fish fat and olive oil respectively, both have very low levels of cholesterol and heart attack because these oils are unsaturated and effectively lower cholesterol and triglyceride levels.

HOW DO WE LOWER OUR BLOOD CHOLESTEROL LEVELS?

You guessed it, by lowering your consumption of saturated fat and cholesterol and eating small amounts of unsaturated fats in accordance with the HealthMark guidelines. This will work for 80 to 85 percent of you. If after 4 to 6 months your blood cholesterol and triglycerides have not reached the desired values, you should consult with a physician to obtain the medication necessary to lower them to optimal levels. The type of medication you may require will depend on the pattern of the abnormality seen on your blood test. Someone with experience in the field of treating these disorders should be consulted.

Make sure, after you have had a blood test, that you get the actual report back so you can assess whether the results are truly normal. Do not accept the interpretation that the tests "are normal; don't worry."

Remember, the only important factor is to have a normal lipid profile. It is the numbers that will determine whether you get heart attack and strokes, so make sure that you get to know your values and then follow them until they normalize. You alone are responsible for this. *Take charge. Know your numbers.*

WHAT HAPPENS IF WE DON'T LOWER OUR CHOLESTEROL LEVELS?

If your cholesterol level, particularly the LDL level, is elevated, you will begin to deposit cholesterol in your arteries until symptoms develop, e.g., heart attacks, strokes, and other symptoms depending on where the blockage is. The higher the LDL, the faster the development. If other risk factors are present—high blood pressure, smoking, diabetes, obesity, elevated triglycerides—the process will be accelerated greatly.

As the cholesterol builds in the arterial wall, it will eventually slow the blood flow enough so that a blood clot forms, totally occluding the artery and resulting in a heart attack or stroke. This will not occur until you have a blockage of 70 percent or more, indicating the presence of far advanced disease. Recent studies have shown that consumption of an aspirin every other day will prevent heart attacks in males. This is because aspirin prevents the blood clot from forming. It does not do anything to delay the progression of cholesterol buildup. Aspirin prevents the blood platelets from adhering together to form blood clots.

The only people who need to take aspirin are those who have risk factors. If you don't have any risk factors and exercise regularly you don't need the aspirin, as exercise can induce similar changes to prevent blood clots from forming. People with high blood pressure should be cautious of aspirin because there is a higher incidence of hemorrhagic strokes (from bleeding) in people who take aspirin regularly. Consult your doctor.

Heart attacks and strokes are not diseases of the heart and brain but of the arteries that supply blood to these organs, the arteries which have been blocked with cholesterol. As mentioned, occasionally, a weakening in the artery wall will form, causing a ballooning or aneurysm, which may rupture with disastrous consequences.

In summary, the natural history of the disease is a relentless progression until some cardiovascular disaster occurs.

WHAT GOOD DOES LOWERING OUR BLOOD CHOLESTEROL LEVELS DO?

Let us look at the evidence from two angles: (1) reducing the risk for heart attack and (2) reversing atherosclerosis.

Reducing the Risk for Heart Attack

There is a magic formula that if you lower your cholesterol 1 percent, you reduce your risk of heart attack by 2 percent. The evidence for this formula is based largely on the Lipid Research

Coronary Prevention trial, perhaps the best trial done to date. A group of men in their late forties, all with very high cholesterol levels, were placed on cholesterol-lowering medication or placebo in a randomized fashion. Those who did not lower their cholesterol levels went on to have heart attacks at the expected high rate. Those who did lower their cholesterol showed this formula: A 9 percent cholesterol drop produced a 19 percent reduction in risk for heart attack, and a 25 percent drop produced a 50 percent reduction in heart attacks.

In other studies where factors influencing progression of atherosclerosis are evaluated in people with documented coronary artery disease, we find that 80 percent of cases usually progress if the lipids are not lowered. In the remaining 20 percent no further progression is seen if lipids are normalized, particularly the cholesterol-HDL ratio.

In addition, people undergoing coronary bypass operations will progress and close off their grafts (80 percent in 8 years) if no change in lipids is achieved, whereas in 20 percent who normalize their lipids and get their cholesterol-HDL ratios below 3.5, no further progression is seen.

It appears that in all these studies the most important factors in limiting progression of atherosclerosis are normalizing lipid values and keeping the cholesterol-HDL ratio at 3.5 or below. Stopping smoking, controlling blood pressure, and diabetes appeared to be less significant, but are nevertheless important.

Reversing Atherosclerosis

We can readily induce atherosclerosis in animals by feeding them diets very high in cholesterol and fat. We can also reverse it completely in the same animals by placing them on low fat, low cholesterol, and high carbohydrate diets to normalize their blood cholesterol levels.

In humans we have had isolated reports of regression (reversal) of atherosclerosis. It was not until June of 1987 that the results of a landmark study by Dr. David Blankenhorn of the University of Southern California were released. For the first time we have a well-controlled regression study. This study was done on a group of men who had previously undergone coronary bypass operations. The results showed that the group that lowered their LDL cholesterol and raised their HDL cholesterol levels were able to stop the progression of atherosclerosis, and 16 percent were able to actually reverse it.

The study group was small. However, it was matched against a similar group of men (control group) who did not lower their blood cholesterol levels and went on to progress in their atherosclerosis at the expected rate. So conclusive was the study that at the end of the 2 years they switched the control group over to the cholesterol-lowering regimen (a combination of diet and medication), as the researchers felt it was unethical to withhold the treatment from them.

What we don't know are all the various factors that influence reversal of atherosclerosis. In the next 5 years we hope to have this information. How do age, length of time you have the disease, severity of individual risk factors, and the combination of risk factors influence regression? These are all questions that must be answered.

Nevertheless, we have enough evidence that indicates normalizing lipid values and the cholesterol-HDL ratio are the most important factors in preventing and reversing atherosclerosis. An advisory panel of the National Institutes of Health has concluded beyond reasonable doubt that "reduction of cholesterol can significantly lower the incidence of heart attack." In fact, the average cholesterol for a person in the United States is 215 mg/dl, and lowering it 10 percent (21.5 mg/dl) will save an additional 100,000 lives annually from heart attacks. We don't even have to reverse atherosclerosis completely, only reduce it to a subcritical level, below 70 percent blockage, in order to achieve great symptomatic improvement and reduce the risk for heart attack or stroke.

Whether you have existing heart disease, vascular disease, or positive cardiac risk factors, the message is the same. By normalizing your lipid values and reversing or controlling all other risk factors, you can stop the progression of cholesterol buildup. In a significant percentage of people reversal or regression of this process will also occur.

We have clear evidence that lowering your blood cholesterol level (particularly the LDL fraction) and raising your HDL level will prevent buildup of cholesterol in arteries, and in some individuals reversal or regression will be seen.

Don't wait for symptoms before you decide to make a change—you may be too late.

T H R E E

The Fats in Our Foods

In the United States today more than half the food we eat is processed. Humans evolved on a diet low in animal protein and rich in complex carbohydrates and fiber. Our new diet, low in fiber and complex carbohydrates and high in fat and cholesterol, is overtaxing our metabolic systems. The resultant breakdowns are in the form of the diseases we have already discussed. Obviously, we need to change the way we eat. Fortunately, the changes are not difficult to make and are the same for all the diseases: a "one-diet, cure-all" program.

Table 3-1 compares the composition of the typical U.S. diet to the HealthMark program.

How far do we have to reduce dietary fat and cholesterol in order to achieve optimal lowering of blood levels of cholesterol and triglyceride?

One school of thought says that any fat and cholesterol intake is bad and should be avoided at all costs. These diets (like the Pritikin diet) usually have 8 to 10 percent of their calories as fat and 50 to 100 mg of cholesterol per day. They all are effective in lowering cholesterol 20 to 25 percent in a 3- to 4-week period. However, a diet that has 8 to 10 percent of its caloric value as fat will serve only minimal amounts of animal protein. Consisting of mostly vegetables, grains, and cereals, it will be unpalatable and unfamiliar

Table 3-1   Typical U.S. Diet and HealthMark Diet

	Typical U.S. Diet	*HealthMark Diet*
Cholesterol consumed (mg)	450–750	150
Percentage of calories eaten as:		
Protein	15–20	10–15
Carbohydrate	40–45	> 65
Fat	40	20
Saturated	15	< 7
Polyunsaturated	7	7
Mono-unsaturated	18	7
Total grams of fat per 2,000-calorie intake		
Total Fat (g)	89	< 45
Saturated	33	< 15
Polyunsaturated	16	15
Mono-unsaturated	40	15

to most. These dietary programs do not produce long-term compliance and therefore are not effective. What good is a diet that you cannot stick with?

THE HEALTHMARK WAY TO REDUCE FAT INTAKE

The HealthMark program offers a more moderate approach. It has been found to produce the same amount of cholesterol and triglyceride lowering as the extreme dietary programs. A higher intake of fats, but with emphasis on the intake of good fats (oils), and a slightly higher intake of cholesterol are permitted. This allows the use of more animal protein and the preparation of foods that look and taste familiar. The HealthMark program provides you with a nutritional program that you can live with for the rest of your life. Diets that are effective for only a short time are useless and may do more harm than good.

Eating correctly most of the time (90 percent) will allow for a little "indiscretion time" (cheats and treats). This is called the "90 percent rule," that is, 10 percent is allowed for treats. Today in the United States the indiscretion has become the rule. We need to change this in order to return to a happier and healthier life.

Ten percent time for treats should be done without guilt. What you cheat on is your pleasure. For me, it is desserts. Many a Health-Mark graduate will delight in catching me eating some scrumptious dessert. I always explain that this is my 10 percent time.

The longer you are on a low fat dietary program, the less tolerant you become of fatty foods. When you do eat a fatty meal, you don't sleep well and the next morning you feel like you have been run over by a truck and your legs don't want to work when you exercise. You realize that the fatty meal was the culprit, and the desire to eat another becomes less and less. It is a wonderful feeling to know that your body works as a finely tuned machine, and thus you do not want to feed it bad fuel. I am stuck with my sweet tooth, and yet I have learned to control it.

The secret to long-term success is learning to climb back up on the wagon. When you go on vacation, for example, and don't exercise and eat as well as you should, no great harm is done if when you return, you resume your regular exercise and eating programs. It will take a few days to clean out the systems and allow your blood levels of cholesterol and triglyceride to return to normal.

As long as your 10 percent times are not too close together, no great harm is done. There is no fixed rule as to what 10 percent time actually means—only that if you do the right thing most of the time, then the little indiscretions don't count. This is a compromise that you have to work out based on keeping the blood levels of cholesterol and triglyceride normal 90 percent of the time. (See Chapter 7 to learn how to gauge how well you are doing.)

HEALTHMARK NUTRITIONAL GUIDELINES

1. Reduce cholesterol intake to 150 milligrams per day.

2. Reduce fat intake to 20 percent of total calories eaten and do not exceed 45 grams of fat per day.

3. Eat more polyunsaturated and mono-unsaturated fats.

4. Eat more fiber, 20 to 30 grams per day.

5. Eat less chemically preserved and artificially colored and flavored food.

6. Reduce alcohol consumption to fewer than two drinks per day.

7. Drink no more than two cups of caffeinated coffee per day.

8. Eat 1 teaspoon or less of salt per day.

9. Have at least two glasses of nonfat or low fat dairy product per day (milk or yogurt).

Let us look at all these recommendations in more detail.

WHAT EXACTLY IS CHOLESTEROL?

What Is It?

Cholesterol is a waxy, fatlike substance that is found only in animal foods. It is not fat. Think of it as wax that is found in all meats, poultry, fish, and dairy products.

How Much Do We Need?

We need very little cholesterol. Essentially, your liver can make as much cholesterol as you need, and whatever you eat is in excess of your daily requirement. At HealthMark we limit intake to 150 milligrams per day. There is no such thing as cholesterol deficiency.

If you never ate another gram of cholesterol, your liver would continue to make all you need.

What Does It Do?

Cholesterol is used in minute amounts by your body to make certain hormones, such as cortisone, estrogen, and testosterone. There are billions of cells in the body, and each cell wall contains some cholesterol.

How Do We Get Rid of It?

There is only one pathway for excretion of cholesterol. It is transported to the liver, and there it is incorporated into bile. The bile is then secreted into the gallbladder, where it is discharged into the intestine in response to eating fat. Bile helps to emulsify fat so that it can be absorbed. As the bile flows down the intestine, most of it will be reabsorbed, and the remainder will be lost in the stool. Bile pigment is what gives the stool its brown color.

We are able to get rid of only small amounts of cholesterol in this way, as we do not increase the amount of bile (cholesterol) excreted to any large degree when we consume large quantities of cholesterol. In fact, the body's production of cholesterol is also not greatly diminished by eating large quantities of it. The overall effect for most of us of eating large quantities of cholesterol is the absorbtion of a significant proportion of cholesterol. The excess is then deposited in your arteries, eventually causing heart attacks and strokes. There is a small percentage of people who can eat lots of cholesterol and fat and never elevate their lipid levels and develop atherosclerosis. These are the people with "good" genes.

Where Do We Find Cholesterol?

Cholesterol is found only in animal foods. Table 3-2 lists the cholesterol content of the commonly eaten foods. It is not found in fruit, vegetables, grains, or cereals.

The foods that are very rich in cholesterol and should be avoided are the organ meats (kidney, liver, sweetbreads, and brains), egg

Table 3-2   Cholesterol Content of Selected Foods

Food	Cholesterol (mg)
Meats (6-oz serving)	
Beef	140–170
Lamb	170
Pork	150
Veal	160–170
Organ Meats (6-oz serving)	
Brains	3492
Kidney	658
Liver	662
Poultry (6-oz serving)	
Chicken, dark	160
Chicken, white	140
Turkey, dark	135
Turkey, white	110
Fish (6-oz serving)	
Clams	53
Crab	100–170
Flounder	74
Haddock	80
Halibut	79
Lobster	163
Mackerel	103
Oysters	81
Salmon, canned	60
Sardines	220
Shrimp	240–300

(continued)

Table 3-2 (*Continued*)

Food	Cholesterol (mg)
Tuna, canned	110
Dairy	
Egg yolk (from large egg)	275
Butter (1 tbsp)	34
Buttermilk (8 oz)	5
Cottage cheese, 4% (8 oz)	48
Cottage cheese, 2% (8 oz)	24
Cheese, cream (1 oz)	31
Cheese, hard (1 oz)	24–28
Cheese, spread (1 oz)	18

yolks, butter, whole milk dairy products, and shrimp. The good news for most of us is that liver is not a nutritious food. A half pound of brains has over 4000 milligrams of cholesterol. Avoiding these foods will eliminate the excess quantities of cholesterol that may be eaten.

If we now control the quantity of animal protein eaten, we can easily control cholesterol intake on a daily basis. Six ounces of animal protein per day (equivalent to two chicken breasts) is all we need for our daily protein requirements. There is very little difference in the cholesterol content of low fat meats, poultry, and fish.

Eating 6 ounces of animal protein per day will keep the daily cholesterol intake at about 150 mgs or less if the other cholesterol-rich foods are avoided. It is almost impossible to eat exactly 6 ounces every day, so we advise you to go without animal protein 1 day a week to make up for the excess that may have been consumed on the other days.

We have heard that we should avoid beef and eat more fish and chicken. Why all this hoopla if the cholesterol difference in these foods is not significant? It is the fat content of meat that makes it less desirable than poultry and fish, but eating low fat meat is comparable to eating chicken.

In addition, eating 6 ounces of fish for lunch and 6 ounces of chicken for dinner is still no good because you may be eating almost 300 milligrams of cholesterol per day (although some fish is low in cholesterol; see Table 3-2).

Avoiding beef and eating only fish and chicken therefore, does not guarantee good cholesterol levels. Eating 6 ounces of low fat animal protein per day will keep your cholesterol intake at a desirable level and will contribute toward keeping your blood cholesterol levels within the optimal range.

Cholesterol intake is easy to control: Eat 6 ounces of animal protein per day and avoid the high-cholesterol foods.

HOW FATS AFFECT CHOLESTEROL LEVELS

Fats are categorized as good or bad based on their effect on the blood cholesterol level. Bad fats obviously raise the blood cholesterol level, whereas good fats tend to lower it.

The bad fats are the saturated fats, and the good fats are unsaturated (the polyunsaturated and mono-unsaturated fats). The typical U.S. diet contains much too much fat (42 percent of the calories), and most of this fat is saturated. What we need to do is reduce our intake of fat to no more than 20 percent of calories eaten or no more than 45 grams per day.

This is achieved by lowering the intake of saturated fats to a minimum and reducing the intake of the unsaturated fats (polyunsaturated and mono-unsaturated). The amount of polyunsaturated fat consumed, however, should be twice the amount of saturated fat consumed. This is called the polyunsaturated-to-saturated-fat ratio or P:S ratio, and it should be at least 2:1. This dietary ratio is important for maximal blood cholesterol lowering.

The maximum amount of fat consumed daily should be less than 45 grams per day, as follows: 15 grams of polyunsaturated fat, 15 grams of mono-unsaturated fat, and less than 15 grams of saturated fat.

Note that 15 grams is 1 tablespoon of fat. Therefore, we should have 1 tablespoon of polyunsaturated fat and 1 tablespoon of monounsaturated fat per day. Keep the intake of saturated fat at less than 1 tablespoon of fat (15 grams) per day, and the less you eat, the better. This does not mean that you should add 1 tablespoon of corn oil (polyunsaturated) and 1 tablespoon of olive oil (monounsaturated) to your diet every day. These oils are already present in the foods you are eating. Thus you use *small* amounts of these types of oils in your food preparation, e.g., in salad dressings, for sautéing, baking, and cooking. Do not add large quantities of oil (even if it is good oil) to your food.

At 9 calories per gram of fat, 45 grams equal 405 calories (9 × 45). If we use a straight 20 percent of calories eaten as fat, this will apply up to a maximum of only 2000 calories per day. If you are consuming more than 2000 calories per day, the limit of 45 grams of fat applies (see Table 3-3).

If we keep the percentage of fat constant and increase the caloric intake as above, the amount of fat consumed becomes erroneous. Competitive athletes consuming this many calories should keep their fat intakes at 45 grams of fat per day no matter what, and the additional calories should come from carbohydrates. Thus an athlete consuming 3000 calories per day will be eating 13 percent of the diet as fat, and most of the calories will come from carbohydrates. At 4000 calories, 45 grams of fat is 10 percent fat, and at 5000 calories, 45 grams is 8 percent fat. By keeping the fat intake constant at 45 grams per day, the actual percentage of fat eaten decreases as the caloric intake increases with the addition of lots of carbohydrates, which an athlete needs.

Table 3-3   Calories and Fat Consumed Daily

Calories per Day	Percentage of Calories Eaten as Fat	Fat (g)
2000	20	45
3000	20	66
4000	20	88
5000	20	111

There are two important concepts to understand in determining the fat content of various foods:

1. *Be aware of the percentage of fat eaten in particular foods:* We know that each gram of fat eaten contains 9 calories, and if we know the total amount of calories present in food and the number of grams of fat, we can calculate the percentage of calories as fat. In low fat yogurt, for example, total calories are 240; fat, in grams, is 3. To convert the grams of fat to calories, we multiply the grams of fat by 9 (9 calories per gram), that is, $3 \times 9 = 27$. Next we divide the calories as fat by the total calories and multiply by 100 to get the percentage of calories as fat.

$$(27 \times 100) \div 240 = 11\% \text{ fat}$$

You should try to keep the fat content of foods eaten at 20 percent of the calories of that food and be aware of the total amount of fat in grams you are eating. The percentage of fat in the yogurt above is good. All foods should be assessed in this fashion to determine whether the particular food falls into the "legal" category.

2. *Always keep an account of the amount of saturated fat eaten:* Foods may be high in saturated fat, but the overall fat content of the food is very low, for example, 1 to 2 grams, and thus it is not all bad. However, many small quantities of saturated fat will mount up during the course of a day. Label reading is therefore extremely important in determining what foods are indeed "healthy."

In Japan and Thailand the intake of fat is less than 45 grams per day, whereas in the United States it is 150 grams per day and in New Zealand 100 grams per day. There is a corresponding high incidence of the "degenerative diseases" in those countries on high fat diets.

Fats are used as a fuel only in the absence of carbohydrates. When used, they burn inefficiently, producing toxic by-products called *ketones* which build up in the body and may cause nausea, fatigue, and apathy. Thus fat is not a desirable fuel source.

Let us look at the three fats in a little more detail.

Saturated Fats: Bad

What Are They?

Saturated fats are the fats that are solid at room temperature.

How Much Do We Need?

There is no known need for saturated fat. The body can manufacture all the saturated fat it needs; therefore, you should eat the least amount of saturated fat possible. We should eat less than 1 tablespoon of this fat per day.

Saturated fat raises the total and the LDL cholesterol levels.

How Do We Get Rid of Them?

Saturated fats, like all fats that are not burned as energy, are stored in the body's fat stores (adipose tissue). The only way we can get rid of fat stores is to burn the fat with exercise. Slightly reduced caloric intake together with a regular aerobic exercise program is the most efficient way to burn fat (see Chapter 6).

Where Do We Find Them?

Saturated fats are found in all animal fats and a few vegetable products (coconut oil, palm oil, cocoa butter, and hydrogenated fats).

Animal sources of saturated fat are all meats (beef, pork, veal, lamb), poultry, and dairy products. The major difference between poultry and meat products is that in poultry the fat is stored in the skin. Thus when you cook chicken or turkey without the skin, you remove most of the fat. The white meat of these products is only

20 percent fat, whereas the dark meat is a little higher. In prime or choice meat products the fat is marbled into the muscle (meat), and therefore they are extremely fatty. When you remove the external fat, the remaining meat is generally 60 to 80 percent fat, that is, 60 to 80 percent of the calories eaten.

When assessing meat products, it is vitally important that you look not only at the amount of fat in grams but also at the percentage of calories as fat. For example, hamburger that is advertised as 88 percent lean is meant to imply that it is a lean product. the 88 percent lean designation means that there is 12 percent fat. Thus there are 12 grams of fat per 100 grams of meat (100 grams equal 3.5 ounces). Thus 100 grams of this hamburger contain approximately 250 calories; therefore, it contains 108 calories from fat (12 times 9). This product now appears to derive 43 percent of its calories from fat, mostly (50 percent) saturated fats. Meats also contain a significant amount of mono-unsaturated fat and a small amount of polyunsaturated fat. Be careful of hamburger bought in the supermarkets or butcher stores as they mix the ground beef with fat. Ground chuck or ground round always has extra fat added to it. It is better to buy the lean cuts from lean beef, trim all the visible fat, and grind it yourself or have the butcher grind it in front of you after trimming all the visible fat (called *zero-trimmed*). Even lean grown meats that may be used for ground beef will have fat added to them. Thus a beef product that may have started out as lean is no longer lean.

There is nothing wrong with beef. In fact, it is a nutritious food, containing vitamin B_{12} and iron, and it is a good source of protein. When the cattle are taken from the range to the feedlots, they are in great shape, weighing about 600 to 700 pounds, and are nice and lean. In the feedlots they are force-fed and given growth hormones, growth stimulants, and antibiotics. By the time they are slaughtered, they weigh about 1100 pounds.

The weight they have gained is mostly in fat. In fact, if you ate the beef when it first arrived in the feedlot before it was force-fed and given all the chemicals, it would be extremely lean. Most cuts would contain 20 to 30 percent or less of their calories as fat, and some cuts would be leaner than chicken or fish.

The "finished beef" usually has 60 to 80 percent of its calories as fat. This is the major difference between poultry and beef or other meat products and is why we are warned to eat fish and poultry instead of meat. If you are able to find grass-fed or range-fed beef or lamb that hasn't been force-fed or given hormones and antibiotics, you can eat this meat as frequently as you want (if it is zero-trimmed).

In Colorado we have a few sources of "natural" low-fat beef available. We have tested these products and found them to be consistently low in fat, as lean as chicken and in some cuts as lean as fish. These products have received the HealthMark endorsement, which means that they have consistently less than 30 percent of their calories as fat and are guaranteed to receive no hormones or antibiotics and will have 10 grams of fat or less in a 6-ounce portion.

It is ironic that the very standards that beef is graded by are the standards that make it the most unhealthy or least desirable. The higher the fat content, the higher the grade of beef. Choice and prime beef are the fattiest. This needs to change, and the grading system should be reversed so that the leanest beef gets the highest grade.

Buffalo is traditionally very lean. Buffalo is grass-fed and is not given any hormones and chemicals; consequently they have as low as 6 percent of calories as fat. Wild game is as lean as buffalo, except for the farm-raised game sold to some restaurants.

Goose and duck are too fatty to be eaten on a regular basis and should be considered as a 10 percent treat. Pheasant and Cornish game hen are lean.

Dairy products are too high in fat if eaten as whole milk products. Hard cheeses are 70 percent fat, and cream cheese is 95 percent fat. The new low fat cream cheese such as Neufchatel and the Philadelphia Kraft are reduced to 70 percent fat and are still too fat to eat on a regular basis.

The cheeses made with part-skim milk, such as the new Kraft Lite, Jarlsberg, mozzarella, Romano, Parmesan, and ricotta cheeses, all have 50 percent of their calories as fat. They are better choices but are still too fatty to eat in large quantities. Small quantities can be eaten, e.g., Parmesan on your pasta or salad, or a cheese sandwich made with a thin slice of low fat cheese, or pizza made with part-skim milk mozzarella cheese.

At first glance this may appear not to conform with HealthMark guidelines. However, if you order thin-crust pizza without extra cheese, pepperoni, or meatballs, you will eliminate most of the additional fat. A pizza eaten with part-skim milk mozzarella cheese and mushrooms, onions, peppers, or any vegetable of your choice will be about 27 to 29 percent of the calories as fat and can be eaten occasionally. Now tell me that is not good news.

Most of milk is water. In whole milk only 4 percent of the volume is fat, but 48 percent of the calories consumed are from fat. Table 3-4 shows what percentage of different types of milk is calories in the form of fat. The best milk products are the ones that are 1 percent fat or less, with the very best being the nonfat products. In fact, the only "legal" cheese made is the 1 percent cottage cheese, which is used as is, or it can be made into fluffy cream cheese: a great base for dips and creamy salad dressings. One percent cottage cheese can be found in Colorado in the generic form or in the Weight Watchers brand.

The vegetable sources of saturated fat are coconut oil and palm oil. You may not think that you eat these commonly. However, when you read the labels of almost all the baked goods and candy you buy, you will find either or both these oils in them. These

Table 3-4   Percentages of Fat as Calories in Milk

Percentage of Fat by Volume	Percentage of Fat as Calories
4% whole milk	48–51
2% milk	35
1% milk	19
Skim milk	4
Nonfat milk	0–3

fats are more saturated than butter and should be avoided. Read labels.

When you treat yourself to a delicious tropical health drink called piña colada, the healthiest part of the drink is the pineapple juice and the alcohol. The coconut juice that is in the drink has 82 percent of its calories as saturated fat. Suddenly this tropical health drink does not look so healthy. If you are fortunate enough to be having this drink in Hawaii or Mexico when you are on vacation, they will serve it to you in a large coconut as you sunbathe by the pool or on the beach. When you are done with the liquid portion of the treat, they will usually cut the coconut up for you to eat. This is not fruit; 75 percent of its calories are saturated fat. Heart of palm salad is all right because the palm oil comes from the seed of the palm, not the heart.

Cocoa butter is also a saturated fat and is used to make chocolate. There is some preliminary evidence that the predominant saturated fatty acid in cocoa butter (stearic acid) does not raise cholesterol levels as much as the other saturated fatty acids. If you are a chocolate lover (like me), it is better to eat the dark chocolate (it's mostly cocoa butter) as the other chocolate is made with milk products. Chocolate should be eaten sparingly and lovingly. We need more evidence before we legalize chocolate.

Hydrogenated fats are another source of saturated fat, including margarines and vegetable shortening. Saturated fat is solid at room temperature, and polyunsaturated fat is liquid at room temperature. When you take a polyunsaturated fat (liquid) such as corn oil or safflower oil and convert it into a solid to make margarine or shortening, you have to hydrogenate it; i.e., add hydrogen atoms to it.

This process of hydrogenation is the same as saturation. You are converting a polyunsaturated fat to a saturated fat. When you read the label of these products, it always tells you that there is no cholesterol. This is correct, inasmuch as vegetable oil never did contain cholesterol. However, these products (margarines and shortenings) do have saturated fat.

In fact the more solid the margarine (stick margarine), the more saturated it is; therefore, the more liquid the margarine, the less saturated it is. The margarines that are in the squeeze bottles or the soft tubs are the best.

Margarine labels now list the amount of polyunsaturated and saturated fat. Look for the P-S ratio. If it is not there, calculate it before deciding that the margarine is okay. The P-S ratio should be greater than 2.5.

Margarines should be used with caution and within the Health-Mark guidelines. Remember, 1 teaspoon of fat has 5 grams of fat, which is 45 calories, and a tablespoon is 15 grams, or 135 calories. This may be 45 or 135 unnecessary calories added to your toast or corn.

Thus far it is not all that bad. I have told you that you can eat the right kind of low fat beef, pizza, chicken, and fish. The only foods that you absolutely have to watch out for are egg yolks, organ meats, and butter. Butter not only has a large amount of cholesterol but has a tremendous amount of saturated fat (65 percent) and should be avoided. An egg yolk contains 275 milligrams of cholesterol and 5 grams of fat (mostly saturated), and thus 45 of its 63 calories are from fat.

Remember that all animal foods (except fish) contain cholesterol and saturated fat and give your blood cholesterol the double whammy. The combination of cholesterol and saturated fat does a wonderful job of raising your blood cholesterol levels. See Tables 3-5 and 3-6 for the saturated fat content of some meats and dairy products.

In contrast to saturated fats, unsaturated fats lower blood cholesterol and triglyceride levels. Unsaturated fats include polyunsaturated and mono-unsaturated fats, and are characterized by being liquid at room temperature.

Polyunsaturated Fats

What Are They?

Polyunsaturated fats are the oils found in vegetables and fish and are liquid at room temperature. The polyunsaturated fatty acids found in vegetable oil are called the *omega-6* fatty acids, and the fatty acids found in fish oil are called the *omega-3* fatty acids.

Table 3-5 Saturated Fat Content of Selected Meats

(All portions are 6 ounces unless otherwise noted.)

	Calories	Protein (g)	Fat (g)	Calories as Fat (%)	Cholesterol (mg)
Beef, feedlot					
Brisket, all grades, L&F	664	39	55	74	158
Brisket, all grades, L	410	49	21	47	158
Chuck, oven roast, L&F	602	45	45	67	168
Chuck, oven roast, L	398	56	17	39	170
Flank, L&F	432	42	28	58	122
Flank, L	414	43	25	55	120
Rib, whole ribs, L&F	626	36	52	75	146
Rib, whole ribs, L	396	44	23	52	138
Short ribs, L&F	800	36	71	80	160
Short ribs, L	502	52	31	55	158
Round, full cut, L&F	466	48	31	59	142
Round, full cut, L	330	43	13	37	140
Bottom round, L&F	448	51	26	52	162
Bottom round, L	382	54	16	40	162
Eye of round, L&F	414	46	25	53	124
Eye of Round, L	312	49	11	33	118
Tip round, L&F	432	45	27	56	140
Tip round, L	328	49	13	36	138
Porterhouse steak, L&F	508	43	36	64	140
Porterhouse steak, L	370	48	18	45	136
T-bone steak, L&F	552	41	42	68	142
T-bone steak, L	364	48	18	44	136

(continued)

Table 3-5   Saturated Fat Content of Selected Meats (*Continued*)

	Calories	Protein (g)	Fat (g)	Calories as Fat (%)	Cholesterol (mg)
Tenderloin, L&F	460	44	30	59	146
Tenderloin, L	352	48	16	42	144
Top loin, L&F	486	43	33	61	136
Top loin, L	352	49	16	41	130
Wedge bone sirloin, L&F	480	47	31	59	144
Wedge bone sirloin, L	360	51	15	38	152
Ground, extra L	434	49	27	54	168
Ground, L	462	42	31	61	148
Ground, regular	492	41	35	64	152
Brains	272	19	21	70	3492
Kidneys	244	43	6	22	658
Liver	274	41	8	27	662
Pancreas	460	46	29	57	N/A
Tongue	482	38	35	66	182
Typical "natural" low fat beef—available in Colorado					
Tenderloin	195	39	5	23	103
Chuck	202	39	5	22	96
Sirloin	193	39	4	20	103
Ribeye	252	38	11	39	114
Eye of round	185	40	4	17	80
Top round	181	39	3	14	82
Lunch meats					
Bologna, 1 slice, 4½ × ⅛ in	88	3	8	82	16
Bacon, 3 slices	276	8	26	86	56

(*continued*)

Table 3-5   Saturated Fat Content of Selected Meats (*Continued*)

	Calories	Protein (g)	Fat (g)	Calories as Fat (%)	Cholesterol (mg)
Corned beef, 3 oz	213	15	16	68	83
Frankfurter, 5 × ½ in	142	5	13	81	27
Beerwurst & salami, 1 slice, 4 × ⅛ in	76	2	6	81	14
Beerwurst & salami, 1 slice, 2¼ × ¹⁄₁₆ in	20	0.7	1.8	80	4
Chicken, light or dark, with skin	420	46	25	54	150
Chicken, light meat, no skin	306	55	8	25	140–160
Chicken, dark meat, no skin	312	50	11	31	160
Turkey, light or dark, with skin	378	54	17	41	110–135
Turkey, light meat, no skin	270	56	4	13	110
Turkey, dark meat, no skin	288	51	9	28	135
Turkey bologna or franks	378	54	17	41	180
Turkey pastrami	204	31	10	42	174
Veal					
Breast, riblet, cutlet (L), leg, loin, rump, shoulder steak	240	34	10	38	169
Leg, rump, shank, shoulder, L & F	366	49	18	44	168
Loin, L & F	402	45	23	51	174
Ribs, L & F	516	44	36	63	174
Breast riblet, L & F	534	28	46	78	174

(continued)

Table 3-5   Saturated Fat Content of Selected Meats (*Continued*)

	Calories	Protein (g)	Fat (g)	Calories as Fat (%)	Cholesterol (mg)
Lamb					
Chop, leg, roast, sirloin chop, L	318	49	12	34	168
Leg, roast, sirloin chop, L & F	474	43	32	61	168
Breast, chop, rib, L & F	576	37	46	72	168
Pork					
Ham, picnic ham, L	366	50	17	41	150
Boston butt roast, chop, loin, shoulder, L	426	48	23	49	150
Boston butt, ground pork, loin picnic shoulder, L & F	618	40	50	72	150
Spareribs, L & F	750	35	66	79	150

Note: Beef products are choice unless otherwise stated. L&F is lean and fat—the cuts are trimmed with a half inch of fat. L is lean only—the cuts are zero-trimmed. All meat products (beef, pork, and lamb) and poultry are cooked unless otherwise stated. The method of cooking is generally broiling. "Natural" low fat beef was tested raw, all in 6-ounce portions. Raw meat tested has a slightly lower fat and cholesterol content than cooked meat. However, the difference is quite clear in the lower fat, calorie, and cholesterol contents. The similarity to poultry is evident in fat and cholesterol content.

Sources: Material used in this table has been adapted from the following: U.S. Department of Agriculture, *Composition of Foods, Raw, Processed, Prepared,* Handbook no. 8-13, August 1986, and Handbook no. 8-5, August 1979; Pennington and Church, *Food Values of Portions Commonly Used, 1985,* 14th ed., Harper & Row, New York, 1985; Adams, C. F., *Nutritive Value of American Foods in Common Units,* Handbook 8-5, U.S. Department of Agriculture, 1975.

Table 3-6   Saturated Fat Content of Selected Dairy Products

Dairy Product	Serving	Calories	Fat (g)	Fat %	Cholesterol (mg)
Butter	1 tsp	36	4.1	100	12
Buttermilk, skim	8 oz	88	0.2	2	2
Buttermilk, low fat	8 oz	99	2.2	20	9
All cheeses, whole milk	1 oz	80–110	7–9	70–75	25–32
Cottage cheese, whole milk	2 oz	54	2.4	40	8
Cottage cheese, 2% low fat	2 oz	45	0.5	10	4
Cottage cheese, dry curd	2 oz	31	0.2	5.8	3
Cream cheese	2 tbsp	99	9.9	90	31
Cream cheese, light	1 oz	60	5	75	—
Cream, half & half	1 tbsp	20	1.7	76	6
Mozzarella, part-skim milk	1 oz	79	4.9	56	15
Neufchatel, part-skim milk	1 oz	74	6.6	80	22
Cream, sour	1 tbsp	26	2.5	86	5
Vegetable shortening	1 tbsp	106	12	100	—
Whipping cream, heavy	1 tbsp	52	5.6	97	21
Whipping cream, light	1 tbsp	44	4.6	94	17
Milk, whole, 3.7% fat	8 oz	157	8.9	51	35
Milk, whole, 3.5% fat	8 oz	150	8.0	48	34
Milk, 2% fat	8 oz	121	4.7	35	18
Milk, 1% fat	8 oz	102	2.6	19	10
Milk, skim	8 oz	86	0.4	4.2	4

(continued)

Table 3-6   Saturated Fat Content of Selected Dairy Products (*Continued*)

Dairy Product	Serving	Calories	Fat (g)	Fat %	Cholesterol (mg)
Yogurt, nonfat	8 oz	110	0	0	0
Yogurt with fruit, 1% fat	8 oz	260	3	10.3	10

Source: U.S. Department of Agriculture, *Composition of Foods, Raw, Processed, Prepared,* Handbook no. 8-13, August 1986, and Handbook no. 8-5, August 1979; Pennington and Church, *Food Values of Portions Commonly Used, 1985,* 14th ed., Harper & Row, New York, 1985; Adams, C. F., *Nutritive Value of American Foods in Common Units,* Handbook 8-5, U.S. Department of Agriculture, 1975.

How Much Do We Need?

These oils are what we call "essential," meaning that our bodies cannot manufacture them, and therefore we need to ingest a certain amount each day. In fact, we need only 1 teaspoon of vegetable oil per day to supply all the essential fatty acids (linoleic and linolenic acids) we need. You need to keep the intake of these oils at 1 tablespoon per day (15 grams).

What Do They Do?

Polyunsaturated fats are necessary for the absorption of fat-soluble vitamins. They also lower blood cholesterol and triglyceride levels, and thus are called "good fats." In addition, they may also raise the level of good or HDL cholesterol. Populations that generally consume a high proportion of polyunsaturated fat have low cholesterol levels and a low incidence of heart attack, e.g., the Japanese and the Eskimos. These people also consume diets low in saturated fat.

Fish oil also lowers triglyceride and cholesterol levels, and it can thin the blood so that it does not easily clot. In fact, some studies have shown that the regular consumption of fish two to three times per week may reduce the incidence of heart attack by 50 percent. This is due mostly to the fact that you are eating fish instead of high fat meat two to three times per week and also, in part, that you are ingesting some fish oil.

These studies were done with people eating fish generally low in fat, such as flounder and sole. The fattier the fish eaten, the more fish oil you get. There is a trade-off, however, between the good effect of the oil and the excess calories eaten. The fish that have the highest content of fish oil are salmon, mackerel, herring, blue fish, trout, and sardines. All fish have the good fish oil. Most fish are less than 15 percent fat, and just eating the fish ensures that you are not eating some high fat meat product. *Don't fry the fish.* Table 3-7 lists the oil and cholesterol content of selected seafood.

How Do We Get Rid of Them?

There is no need to get rid of polyunsaturated fats and no mechanism other than burning fat, as mentioned above.

Can Excess Amounts Be Harmful?

Yes. Indiscriminate use of large amounts of polyunsaturated fat will cause some potentially harmful problems. Some people have thought that because they lower the levels of cholesterol and triglyceride in the blood, they can eat as much as it takes to keep these levels normal, despite a diet high in fat and cholesterol. Unfortunately, life is not so simple.

Consumption of polyunsaturated fat in large quantities has been associated with a higher incidence of colon cancer, gallstones, obesity, and increased vitamin E requirements. Therefore, we cannot consume large amounts of polyunsaturated fat and should keep within the HealthMark guidelines.

Where Do We Find Them?

Polyunsaturated fats are found in all vegetables, grains, cereals, (*omega-6* fatty acids), and fish (*omega-3* fatty acids). All vegetables, grains, and cereals are low in fat (which is mostly polyunsaturated) and therefore have few calories. We can eat larger quantities of

Table 3-7 Oil and Cholesterol Content of Selected Seafood

Type	Total Fat (g)	Cholesterol (mg)
Fish (6-oz serving)		
Bass, striped	4–0	—
Bluefish	11	101
Catfish	5	101
Cod	11	128
Flounder	2–0	74
Halibut, Pacific	4.0	79
Halibut, Greenland	23	55
Herring, Pacific	24	79
Herring, Atlantic	15	132
Mackerel	24	103
Perch, Ocean	4.6	137
Pike, Northern	11	137
Pike, Walleye	2.0	67
Pompano, Florida	16	147
Red snapper	2.0	—
Sablefish	26	86
Salmon, Atlantic	9.3	84
Salmon, Chinook	18	60
Salmon, coho	10.3	60
Salmon, pink	6.0	60
Salmon, Sockeye	15.0	60
Shark	3.2	75
Sole	2.0	86
Swordfish	4.0	67

(continued)

Table 3-7 Oil and Cholesterol Content of Selected Seafood
(*Continued*)

Type	Total Fat (g)	Cholesterol (mg)
Trout, brook	5.0	116
Trout, lake	17	82
Trout, rainbow	10	98
Tuna, albacore	8	93
White fish, lake	16	103
Crustaceans (6-oz serving)		
Crab, Alaska King	1.3	—
Crab, Dungeness	1.7	101
Crayfish	2.4	270
Lobster	1.5	163
Shrimp, Atlantic brown	2.5	243
Shrimp, Atlantic white	2.5	312
Mollusks (6-oz serving)		
Abalone, New Zealand	1.7	—
Clam, hardshell	1.0	53
Clam, littleneck	1.3	—
Clam, softshell	3.4	—
Conch	4.6	241
Mussel, blue	3.7	68
Octopus	1.7	—
Oyster, eastern	4.3	81
Scallops	1.4	63
Squid	1.9	—

Source: *"The USDA HNIS Provisional Table on the Fatty Acids and Fat Components of Selected Foods, November 1985," Journal of the American Dietetic Association*, June 1986, vol. 86, no. 6, pp. 10–14.

these foods for fewer calories than foods high in fat, which are more dense in calories.

Oatmeal and oat bran (the fiber of oats) are particularly good foods. They contain some polyunsaturated fat, but more important, they contain soluble fiber. This fiber will bind bile (cholesterol) in the intestine and pull it out of the body, and it has definite cholesterol-lowering properties. This same soluble fiber is also found in legumes (beans and peas) and fruit containing pectin.

Potatoes are very low in fat (1 percent) if eaten baked or boiled without any fat added to them in the form of butter or cream. A medium-sized baked potato has only 70 calories, whereas the same potato as french fries has 240 calories. If this is not bad enough, the same potato as potato chips has 440 calories. When you add fat to a food as you do with frying, you add plenty of calories. Most fast-food chains will also fry your french fries, chicken, and fish in beef fat, lard, or hydrogenated vegetable oils.

Mono-unsaturated Fats

What Are They?

Mono-unsaturated fats are the *omega*-9 fatty acids found predominantly in nuts, avocados, and olives.

How Much Do We Need?

We don't need any mono-unsaturated fat as the body can manufacture all it needs from other sources. Keep the intake to 15 grams (1 tablespoon) per day.

What Do They Do?

Mono-unsaturated fats cause a lowering of the blood cholesterol and triglyceride levels, as do the polyunsaturated fats.

Where Do We Find Them?

Unlike the foods that contain polyunsaturated fat (grains, cereals, vegetables, and fruit which have generally less than 10 percent of their calories as fat and are thus low calorie foods), the foods with mono-unsaturated fat (olives, nuts, and avocados) are very high in fat (70 to 80 percent of calories) and thus contain lots of calories: good fat, bad calories. The only nut that is low in fat is the chestnut.

Olive oil is a very good and safe oil to use. The Italian and Greek people in Europe living in the smaller villages (where the diets are less Westernized and more traditional) use a lot of olive oil and have low cholesterol levels and a correspondingly low incidence of heart attack. Olive is a good oil to use in sautéing food and in salad dressings.

Mono-unsaturated fats are also found in most foods that contain some fat; however, the richest sources are those listed above.

Can Excess Be Harmful?

There are no specific harmful effects attributed to monounsaturated fat per se. Because it is ordinarily manufactured by the body, some believe that the ingestion of these oils is potentially less harmful than polyunsaturated fats which are not manufactured by the body and therefore may be considered foreign substances. Table 3-8 shows the fatty composition of oils and fats.

What Is Lecithin?

Lecithin is a substance that is derived from soybean. It is an emulsifier and is claimed to render fat and cholesterol harmless. Lecithin is naturally made in the liver. The lecithin you ingest is digested by the acid in the stomach and never gets absorbed; thus supplements are of no value. There is a myth that the lecithin in egg yolks counteracts the effect of the cholesterol.

SUMMARY

1. Why don't we eat all the polyunsaturated and monounsaturated fat possible and consume a diet high in saturated fat and cholesterol, hoping that this will cause a

Table 3-8   Oils and Fats as Percentage of Total Fatty Acids

Type of Oil	Saturated	Mono-unsaturated	Polyunsaturated
Safflower	9	13	78
Sunflower	11	20	69
Corn	13	25	62
Olive	14	77	9
Soybean	15	24	61
Peanut	18	48	34
Cottonseed	27	19	54
Puritan (canola oil)	7	65	28
Lard	41	47	12
Palm	51	39	10
Beef tallow	52	44	4
Butter fat	66	30	4
Palm kernel	86	12	2
Coconut	92	6	2
Chicken fat	31	47	22

lowering of the blood lipid levels? Saturated fat is twice as potent in raising the blood cholesterol level as an equivalent amount of polyunsaturated fat is in lowering it.

2. Eating large amounts of polyunsaturated and mono-unsaturated fat may have the inherent dangers of consumption of too much of the fats listed below.

3. Eliminating fat altogether does not produce any greater lowering of blood cholesterol levels and produces a diet that is unpalatable and difficult to adhere to.

4. We need a diet that is low enough in fat to produce the cholesterol and triglyceride lowering that is necessary. This diet needs to have a balance of fat so as to have a P-S ratio of 2 to 1 and enough fat to produce familiar-appearing and -tasting food that has 45 grams of fat a day or less. Table 3-9 shows the primary fat content of foods.

Table 3-9   Primary Fat Content of Selected Foods

Saturated	Mono-unsaturated	Polyunsaturated
Butter	Avocado	Almonds
Cheese	Chives	Filberts
Chocolate	Cashews	Fish
Coconut	Peanut	Some margarine
Egg yolk	Peanut hull	Some "lite" mayonnaise
Red meats	Olives	Walnuts
Milk		Grains
Poultry (skin)		Cereals
Vegetable shortening		Vegetables
Mayonnaise		Fruits
Palm oil		

F O U R

Nutritional Building Blocks

PROTEIN: THE MYTHS VERSUS THE FACTS

There is a myth that protein is our most important nutrient. Although it is indeed an essential nutrient, if eaten in excess, it can cause harm. Protein has been packaged, stuffed, and added to every conceivable thing we eat and use from food to shampoo.

What Is It?

Protein is made up of building blocks called *amino acids* (molecules that contain nitrogen). Strings of amino acids form proteins. There are 24 amino acids, and we can manufacture 13 of them from the foods we commonly eat. The other 9 need to be obtained from the diet and are called *essential amino acids*.

Plants and animals incorporate nitrogen from the air and soil into amino acids. Humans cannot do this and must obtain them from the plants and animals they eat. Most animal proteins contain the essential amino acids, whereas the plant proteins are deficient in some. Thus we must use a variety of plant proteins to cover our needs. Vegetarians need to combine foods to provide the full complement of amino acids, especially with grains and legumes (beans and peas), to fulfill daily protein requirements.

There is only one vegetable that is a complete protein. It is a grain originally discovered in South America called quinoa (pro-nounced *keenwa*) and is rapidly becoming popular in the United States.

What Is It Used For?

Proteins make up the building blocks for much of the vital struc-tures of the body and for the enzymes that allow the body to op-erate. The body's proteins are in a constant state of flux and need to be replaced regularly.

When protein is eaten, it is digested and broken down into its basic amino acids, which enter the blood and are distributed to all cells of the body. There is a dynamic breakdown and rebuilding process in the cells of the body for which the protein is necessary.

Protein is not normally used as a fuel source and is used only if not enough calories are supplied by the diet, that is, in very low calorie diets where protein is used as fuel rather than fat and mus-cle mass (protein) rather than fat stores is lost.

How Much Do We Need?

Protein is not stored and therefore should be supplied con-stantly. We need 0.8 grams of protein per kilogram of body weight. An average-size male weighing 70 kilograms (152 pounds) needs only 56 grams of protein per day, and a 50-kilogram (112-pound) woman needs 40 grams per day.

Six ounces of animal protein per day will supply almost all the protein needs. The remainder will come from the other foods we eat. It does not matter whether you are training for triathlons or marathons, walking a few miles a day, or are completely sedentary—your protein needs are almost the same. There is no need to in-crease your protein intake with increased levels of exercise. There is a common misconception among weight lifters and bodybuilders that more protein is needed to build up muscle bulk. This is not supported by any of the current medical literature. Muscle bulk is built from weight lifting, not from eating protein.

What Are the Dangers of Eating Protein in Excess?

When protein is broken down, uric acid and urea (ammonia) are released as by-products. If they remain in the body for a prolonged period, you will become extremely toxic from the urea and may get gout and kidney stones from the uric acid buildup. It is the kidneys' job to excrete these toxins, and the kidneys will take a large amount of fluids from all parts of the body to flush them out. This can place an enormous strain on the kidneys. Some reports have linked chronic kidney damage and failure to excessive protein intake.

Excess protein intake has been shown to cause a loss of calcium in the urine which results from a leaching of calcium from the bones, the major storage sites for calcium. This may be a significant cause of osteoporosis in the United States, where protein is consumed in excess.

We also have to look at what protein is packaged with to assess other harmful effects. This applies to animal proteins, where we find a large amount of animal fat as the major constituent of the foods we readily regard as "good" sources of protein. Most animal proteins are filled with bad animal fat, with the exception of poultry (low in fat) and fish (omega-3 fatty acids).

Protein is a good and necessary nutrient. As in all things, however, too much of a good thing is bad for you.

CARBOHYDRATES: JET FUEL FOR THE BODY

What Are They?

Carbohydrates exist in a few different forms. There are the simple carbohydrates such as sugar, the complex carbohydrates, starches (many sugar molecules together), and fiber (similar to starch but not digestible by the human body).

What Do They Do?

Carbohydrates in any form are the body's main source of energy. After digestion and absorption all carbohydrates are broken down into simple sugars and finally glucose, which is the primary fuel source of the body. Carbohydrates burn cleanly and completely without the production of any toxic by-products; i.e., they are a clean fuel.

Carbohydrate is *jet fuel* and, in fact, is the favorite fuel source of the body. Fat and protein may be burned for energy by the body, but they both produce toxic by-products which interfere with the smooth functioning of the body.

As we become more active, the body's requirement for carbohydrates increases, the exercising muscles thriving on glycogen (sugar). Athletes on high carbohydrate diets have much greater endurance than athletes on a high protein or mixed (carbohydrate and protein) diet. This has led to the concept of carbohydrate loading prior to endurance events. Pasta has become the favorite prerace meal. People around the world who are known for their incredible endurance are known to eat 70 to 80 percent of their diet as complex carbohydrates, e.g., the Nepalese porters and the Tarahumara Indians.

How Much Do We Need?

In the absence of carbohydrates the body will burn fat and protein for energy, which it does less efficiently and with the formation of toxic by-products. Sixty to sixty-five percent of the total daily caloric intake should be carbohydrates. Athletes in training require more daily carbohydrates to replenish the muscular glycogen stores (stored carbohydrate). If this is not done, the lack of muscle glycogen will lead to fatigue, overtraining, and subsequent injury.

During exercise the body will use mainly glycogen, but with regular exercise and training it learns to burn fat, with the benefit of sparing glycogen to allow us greater endurance and allowing us to lose weight.

Most Americans are consuming 45 percent of their calories as carbohydrates, mostly as simple sugars. In fact, most of us will consume almost our own weight in sugar every year.

There is basically no restriction on the amount of carbohydrates eaten, *providing* you are not eating in excess of your daily caloric needs and you are eating complex carbohydrates. Eating any food in excess of your daily caloric requirements will cause the excess calories to be converted into fat (triglycerides). As you may recall from the previous chapter, when triglycerides are formed, they are packaged into a lipoprotein called VLDL. This contains mostly triglyceride but also a small amount of cholesterol. The formation of VLDL by the liver causes production of cholesterol and thus will raise the blood cholesterol level.

Eat only the calories necessary to maintain your ideal weight.

Simple Sugars

The myth about simple sugars is that they are *quick energy*. These sugars are all foods ending in *-ose*, for example, glucose (blood sugar), sucrose (table sugar), maltose, galactose, dextrose, and fructose (fruit sugar). Honey and molasses are sugars and have no added benefit. Brown sugar, turbinado sugar, and "natural sugar" are basically sugars with more sugar (molasses) added to them. Sugar in beets and sugarcane are natural sugars, and yet they do not contain much more than plain sugar and have no added benefits.

The body has no need for sugar other than what it obtains from other carbohydrates such as fruit, vegetables, and grains. Complex carbohydrates are converted into simple sugars for energy. At the turn of the century Americans consumed 27 pounds of sugar per person annually; today they consume about 110 to 130 pounds per person annually.

When we eat a simple sugar, it is immediately absorbed from the stomach and intestine and dumped into the bloodstream. This causes a peak in blood sugar in 30 to 40 minutes, which will in turn cause the pancreas to produce insulin, needed to drive the sugar into the cells of the body. In some of us there is a surplus of insulin production that causes the blood sugar to fall too rapidly to a below normal level. This is called *hypoglycemia*. At this point you get nervous, tremulous, hungry, sweaty, irritable, and you crave more sugar to get rid of the symptoms. This leads to massive swings in the blood sugar levels and also massive mood swings, like riding an emotional roller coaster. Hypoglycemia is not a disease. It is a reaction to eating simple sugars for some people who are more sensitive than others.

Hypoglycemia is easily controlled by eating a balanced diet and consuming complex rather than simple carbohydrates (sugars). The release of sugar from complex carbohydrates is very slow because complex carbohydrates have to be broken down and digested before the sugar is absorbed from the intestine. Compare eating an apple with drinking apple juice. The juice is simple sugar and will be absorbed immediately, whereas the apple needs to be chewed, digested, and absorbed before the sugar is released.

Sugar promotes tooth decay, obesity, and, possibly, diabetes and heart disease.

Complex Carbohydrates

Complex carbohydrates are starchy foods in their natural state. When eaten in their unrefined or natural state, they are all excellent sources of fiber, vitamins, and minerals. If eaten in adequate amounts, they make it unnecessary to take vitamin, mineral, and fiber supplements.

Fruits and vegetables are mostly carbohydrate with small amounts of protein and fat (mostly polyunsaturated). They contain lots of fiber, vitamins, minerals, and water. The sugar in fruit is fructose, and because sugar is packaged in the fiber of the fruit, it has to be broken down before it is released. No hypoglycemia is experienced when eating fruit. Legumes (beans and peas) are good sources of protein in addition to being excellent sources of carbohydrate and soluble fiber.

Nuts provide good sources of carbohydrate and protein as well as fiber, vitamins, and minerals. Nuts are also very high in fat (mostly monounsaturated) and thus contain lots of calories. The only nut that is low in fat is the chestnut, which is 6 percent fat. The other nuts are all 70 to 80 percent fat.

Cereals are great sources of carbohydrate and fiber. Rolled oats (oatmeal) and oat bran (the fiber of oats) are rich sources of carbohydrate and soluble fiber. Instant hot cereals are usually filled with preservatives, sugar, salt, and hydrogenated fats. Unfortunately, to eat a good bowl of hot cereal (oatmeal or oat bran), you must cook it and make the pot dirty.

Because of the cholesterol-lowering properties of the soluble fiber in oats and the polyunsaturated fat, vitamins, and minerals, we can truly say: *Oatmeal or oat bran is the breakfast of champions.* Many dry cereals are excellent breakfast foods because they are rich sources of fiber and carbohydrate. Many of these cereals are filled with salt, sugar, and hydrogenated fats; please read the labels and avoid the ones that contain them.

Granola is often thought to be synonymous with health food but is in fact one of the most unhealthy. It usually contains coconut and coconut oil, which makes it full of saturated fat. It also contains lots of other nuts and sugars (honey), making it a very high calorie breakfast.

Wheat and rice have plenty of carbohydrate, vitamins, minerals, and fiber. When refined into white flour and white rice, the bran (fiber coverings) and germ are removed, leaving only starch, which is simply a string of sugar molecules banded together. This is now no better than eating sugar, empty calories devoid of the much-needed vitamins, minerals, and fiber. Enriched flours replace only 4 of the 26 vitamins removed. Bleaching flour removes all the vitamin E. Use a whole wheat flour or a mixture of whole wheat and unbleached flour. Go for the whole wheat or whole grain products and the brown rice or wild rice.

Fiber

The United States is on a fiber kick in the 1980s and justifiably so. In the 1970s Dr. Dennis Burkitt, a renowned British researcher, reported that people living on high fiber diets had a much lower incidence of colon cancer, diverticulosis, and appendicitis. Fiber is thought to play a significant role in the prevention of these diseases.

Bran (wheat fiber) is added to a variety of foods; however, the fiber present in all fruits, vegetables, cereals, and grains is more than adequate to supply your daily requirements without the need for supplements.

What Is Fiber?

Fiber is the nondigestible parts of the fruits, vegetables, cereals, and grains we eat. Fiber is what gives plants substance, i.e., their structure and stability. Fiber is found only in plants and is found in soluble and insoluble forms (whether or not it is soluble in water).

Where Is Insoluble Fiber Found?

Insoluble fiber is found mostly in grains and cereals. These fibers are insoluble in water, but they are able to absorb several times their own weight in water. This fiber is called the "rotor rooter fiber" because it forms bulk in the intestine and aids in fecal elimination. It causes you to have looser and bulkier bowel movements. The insoluble fibers are cellulose, hemicellulose, and lignin.

Where Is Soluble Fiber Found?

Soluble fiber is found in fruits, vegetables, legumes, and oats. They are water soluble and thicken out in cooking water. This fiber binds bile (cholesterol) in the intestine and helps lower blood cholesterol levels. The soluble fibers are pectins, gums, and mucilages.

In general it is best to consume fibers as a part of the food rather than as an additive or supplement.

What Are the Benefits of Fiber?

1. Fiber passes undigested through the intestine where it forms bulk. In the colon (large intestine) it absorbs a large amount of water, and the result is a bulkier and softer stool.

   Fiber is beneficial in treating and preventing chronic intestinal diseases, such as diverticulosis, spastic colon (nervous bowels), constipation, and hemorrhoids, as well as in the prevention of colon cancer and appendicitis. If bran is used, it should be coarse (cellulose). Finely ground bran may be constipating. A commonly used bulk laxative, metamucil, is hemicellulose and gum and has soluble and insoluble fibers. It may lower cholesterol, as does oat bran. Adequate amounts of water are essential to having soft, bulky stools.

2. Fiber also adds bulk to food and gives a feeling of satiety (fullness) without many calories. For example, apples give a greater feeling of satiety than an equivalent amount of apple sauce, helping to curb the appetite.

3. Both soluble and insoluble fibers increase the sensitivity of the body's cells to insulin and thus help to control diabetes. Fiber also appears to slow the conversion of starch to sugar and reduces the need for insulin.

4. Soluble fiber has been shown to have a definite lowering effect on the blood cholesterol levels. Oat bran or oatmeal, if eaten in large quantities, has been shown to lower cholesterol levels in the blood by as much as 13 to 23 percent. The highest sources of soluble fiber are in oats, oat bran, and legumes (beans and peas).

What Are the Side Effects?

Flatulence and bloating are temporary and usually subside in 3 weeks to 2 months. Excessive amounts of bran supplements have been shown to cause bowel obstruction and can aggravate symptoms in patients with colitis (inflammation of the bowel). When you start the HealthMark program, you will notice more intestinal gas, and you will begin to have two to three loose bowel movements per day (this is normal).

How Much Fiber Do We Need?

We need 20 to 30 grams of fiber per day. A bowl of good high fiber cereal has about 9 to 12 grams of fiber. If you eat a salad, one serving of vegetables and whole grain breads, a bowl of cereal, and two to four fruits daily, then you will easily cover your fiber needs (see Table 4-1).

VITAMINS: DO WE REALLY NEED SUPPLEMENTS?

Vitamins are organic substances essential to human life. They cannot be made by the body and must be provided by the diet. Their functions are varied. When vitamin deficiencies occur, specific symptoms result.

The recommended daily allowances (RDAs) for vitamins will provide enough to prevent deficiencies from occurring with a good safety margin. Vitamin deficiencies occur almost only in the third world where people are malnourished.

Certain events influence the body's need for additional vitamins: pregnancy, alcoholism, smoking, illness, and possibly age. A well-balanced diet should require no further vitamin supplementation, but a diet consisting of highly processed foods (the typical U.S. diet) may need vitamin supplements.

The aim is to improve dietary habits rather than take vitamin supplements.

The 13 known vitamins are divided into the fat-soluble and water-soluble vitamins. The fat-soluble ones (A, D, E, and K) are consumed with fat eaten in the diet and are stored in the body. The water-soluble vitamins (B and C) are not stored in the body to any great degree and need to be consumed daily.

General Guidelines

1. Eat whole grains rather than refined flours (whole wheat flour and bread and brown rice.)

2. Use fresh or frozen fruit and vegetables—canning destroys the vitamins.

(continues on page 102)

Table 4-1   The Fiber Content of Selected Foods

Type of Food	Serving	Fiber Content (grams per serving)
Breakfast cereals		
All-Bran	1 cup	25
Bran Buds	1 cup	24
Cheerios	1 cup	1.0
Corn Flakes	1 cup	0.3
Grape-Nuts	1 cup	5.6
Nutri-Grain cereals	1 cup	2.6
Oat Bran, dry	⅓ cup	4.2
Oatmeal, regular quick and instant cooked	1 cup	2.1
100% Bran	1 cup	16.8
Raisin Bran	1 cup	5.3
Rice Krispies	1 cup	0.1
Shredded Wheat	1 cup	3.9
Special K	1 cup	0.2
Total	1 cup	2.0
Wheaties	1 cup	2.0
Fruits		
Apple, with skin	1 medium	3.5
Apricot, fresh	1 medium	0.6
Apricot, dried	5 halves	1.4
Banana	1 medium	2.4
Blueberries	½ cup	2.0
Cantaloupe	¼ melon	1.0
Berries, sweet	10	1.2

(continued)

Table 4-1   The Fiber Content of Selected Foods (*Continued*)

Type of Food	Serving	Fiber Content (grams per serving)
Dates	3	1.9
Grapefruit	½	1.6
Grapes	20	0.6
Orange	1	2.6
Peach, with skin	1	1.9
Pear, with skin	1	6.2
Pineapple	½ cup	1.1
Plums	5	0.9
Prunes	3	3.0
Raisins	¼ cup	3.1
Raspberries	½ cup	3.1
Strawberries	1 cup	3.0
Watermelon	1 cup	0.4
Vegetables (cooked)		
Asparagus, cut	½ cup	1.0
Beans, string	½ cup	1.6
Broccoli	½ cup	2.2
Brussels sprouts	½ cup	2.3
Cabbage, red and white	½ cup	1.4
Carrots	½ cup	2.3
Cauliflower	½ cup	1.1
Peas	½ cup	3.6
Potato, without skin	1 medium	1.4
Potato, with skin	1 medium	2.5
Spinach	½ cup	2.1

(*continued*)

Table 4-1   The Fiber Content of Selected Foods (*Continued*)

Type of Food	Serving	Fiber Content (grams per serving)
Squash	½ cup	1.4
Sweet potatoes	½ medium	1.7
Zucchini	½ cup	1.8
Vegetables (raw)		
Bean sprouts	½ cup	1.5
Celery, diced	½ cup	1.1
Cucumber	½ cup	0.4
Lettuce, sliced	1 cup	0.9
Mushrooms, sliced	½ cup	0.9
Onions, sliced	½ cup	0.8
Pepper, green, sliced	½ cup	0.5
Spinach	1 cup	1.2
Tomato	1 medium	1.5
Legumes		
Baked beans	½ cup	8.8
Kidney beans, cooked	½ cup	7.3
Lentils, cooked	½ cup	3.7
Lima beans	½ cup	4.5
Navy beans, cooked	½ cup	6.0
Breads		
Bagels	1	0.6
Bran muffins	1	2.5
Cracked wheat bread	1 slice	1.0
French bread	1 slice	1.0
Graham crackers	2 squares	2.8

(*continued*)

Table 4-1   The Fiber Content of Selected Foods (*Continued*)

Type of Food	Serving	Fiber Content (grams per serving)
Italian bread	1 slice	0.7
Mixed grain bread	1 slice	0.9
Pumpernickel bread	1 slice	1.9
Raisin bread	1 slice	0.6
White bread	1 slice	0.6
Whole wheat bread	1 slice	1.4
Pasta and rice, cooked		
Macaroni	1 cup	1.0
Rice, brown	1 cup	2.0
Rice, white	1 cup	0.4
Spaghetti, regular	1 cup	1.1
Spaghetti, whole wheat	1 cup	3.9
Nuts		
Almonds	10 nuts	1.1
Filberts	10 nuts	0.8
Peanuts	10 nuts	1.4

Note: The following foods are also rich in soluble fiber: oats and oat bran; fruit with pectin, e.g., apples, bananas, apricots; legumes and barley; black-eyed peas; chick peas; peas; beans, kidney and pinto; dried figs and dried prunes; wheat germ; and whole cornmeal.

Source: *Journal of the American Dietetic Association,* June 1986, vol. 86, no. 6, pp. 738–739. Provisional dietary fiber table USDA.

3. Do not store food for long. One to two days in the refrigerator will cause considerable loss of vitamins. Frozen fruits and vegetables are good because they are picked ripe and frozen immediately, whereas weeks may go by before fresh produce is consumed.

4. Fruit and vegetables should ripen on the plant and in the sun to retain the vitamin C. To preserve the vitamin C, picked fruit should be chilled in a dark place until eaten.

5. Do not soak vegetables.

6. Prepare salad just before eating.

7. Keep all fresh-cut and cooked foods well wrapped in the refrigerator.

8. Pressure cooking, steaming, and microwaving are better than boiling. If you are going to boil food, use as little water as possible.

9. Toasting bread destroys the B vitamins.

Fat-Soluble Vitamins

Vitamin A

Sources: In animal foods, preformed vitamin A is found in liver, eggs, cheese, and butter, which are all very high sources of saturated fat and cholesterol. Plant foods contain carotene, a yellow substance that is converted into vitamin A. It is found in all yellow and dark-green vegetables, e.g., carrots, squash, pumpkin, spinach, dark lettuce, brussels sprouts, and broccoli. These are much healthier sources of vitamin A than the high animal sources.

Daily requirements: Your diet can supply a sufficient quantity of vitamin A. If consumed as a supplement, no more than 10,000 units per day should be taken.

Functions: Vitamin A assists in the formation of healthy skin, hair, mucus membranes, and night vision. Vitamin A is also needed for bone growth and development and reproduction.

Deficiency: Insufficient vitamin A causes night blindness, rough skin, dry eyes, and impaired hair and nail growth.

Overuse symptoms: Overconsumption of vitamin A can produce blurred vision, loss of appetite, headaches, skin rashes, nausea, diarrhea, fatigue, joint pains, liver damage, and insomnia. Ingestion of too much carotene will cause a harmless yellow coloring of the skin called *carotenemia*.

Advantages: Carotene has a cancer-protecting effect (it is an antioxidant).

Vitamin D

Sources: Adequate amounts of vitamin D are made in skin exposed to sunlight. Fortified dairy products, eggs, liver, tuna, salmon, and cod liver oil all contain vitamin D.

Function: Vitamin D aids in the formation and maintenance of bones and teeth as well as in the absorption of calcium and phosphorous.

Deficiency symptoms: Insufficient vitamin D causes rickets in children and osteoporosis in adults.

Overuse symptoms: Too much vitamin D causes calcium deposits all over the body, deafness, nausea, loss of appetite, kidney stones, high blood pressure, high cholesterol, and increased lead absorption.

Vitamin K

Sources: Vitamin K is in green leafy vegetables, cabbage, cauliflower, peas, potato, liver, and cereals and is manufactured by intestinal bacteria (except in the newborn).

Function: Vitamin K is needed for blood clotting and bone metabolism.

Deficiency: A deficiency of vitamin K causes bleeding tendencies and bone loss.

Overuse: Too much vitamin K can produce jaundice in infants; no ill effects have been reported in adults.

Vitamin E

Sources: Vitamin E is found in vegetable oils, margarine, wheat germ, whole grain cereals, liver, dried beans, and green leafy vegetables.

Function: Vitamin E aids in formation of red blood cells, muscles, and other tissues; it protects vitamin A and essential fatty acids from oxidation.

Deficiency: Deficiencies of vitamin E have not been seen in humans.

Overuse: Nothing is definite about overuse of this vitamin; some possible effects are headaches, blurred vision, fatigue, and muscle weakness.

Water-Soluble Vitamins

In general water-soluble vitamins are interdependent, and an increase in one will cause an increase in the need for the others. A high carbohydrate diet will increase the requirements for them because they are needed for carbohydrate metabolism. These vitamins are easily obtained through the diet as long as unrefined foods are eaten.

Vitamin B_1—Thiamine

Sources: Pork, liver, oysters, grains, pasta, bread, wheat germ, oatmeal, peas, and lima beans contain vitamin B_1.

Function: Vitamin B_1 helps release energy from carbohydrates and aids in the synthesis of a chemical in the brain called serotonin.

Deficiency: Insufficient B_1 causes beriberi—a disorder characterized by confusion, weakness, muscle cramps, and an enlarged heart with heart failure.

Overuse: No overuse effects are known at present.

Vitamin B₂—Riboflavin

Sources: Liver, meats, eggs, dark-green vegetables, and cereals contain vitamin B_2.

Function: B_2 helps to release energy from carbohydrates.

Deficiency: Insufficient B_2 causes skin disorders, cracked lips and mouth, and photophobia (extreme light sensitivity).

Overuse: No side effects of too much B_2 are known at present.

Vitamin B₃—Nicotinic Acid or Niacin

Sources: Vitamin B_3 is found in liver, poultry, meat, tuna, eggs, cereals, nuts, peas, grains, and beans. The body can also convert tryptophan to niacin.

Function: Niacin helps release energy from carbohydrates.

Deficiency: A deficiency of B_3 causes pellagra—a skin disorder with diarrhea, confusion, and swelling of the mouth and tongue.

Overuse: Too much B_3 produces duodenal ulcers, liver dysfunction, elevated blood sugars, and gout.

Other advantages: In massive doses niacin is an effective medication to lower blood cholesterol. Because of its side effects, it should never be used without the supervision of a physician.

Vitamin B₆—Pyridoxine

Sources: Vitamin B_6 is in whole grains, cereals, liver, avocados, spinach, green beans, bananas, poultry, meat, nuts, potatoes, and green leafy vegetables.

Function: Vitamin B_6 aids in the absorption and metabolism of proteins. It also helps the body use fats and form red blood cells.

Deficiency: Insufficient B_6 causes skin disorders, cracked mouth, smooth tongue, confusion, nausea, dizziness, and kidney stones. Oral contraceptives and high protein diets increase the need for pyridoxine.

Overuse: Too much B_6 causes confusion, paralysis, and coma. Recently, vitamin B_6 has been used in high doses in the treatment of premenstrual syndrome where these side effects were first noted. It should be used with extreme caution, if at all.

Vitamin B_{12}—Cobalamin

Sources: Vitamin B_{12} is found in animal foods only—liver, kidney, fish, eggs, meat, and oysters.

Function: This vitamin is used in the formation of red blood cells and the nervous system.

Deficiency: Insufficient B_{12} can be linked with pernicious anemia, which is associated with nervous system dysfunction characterized by loss of sensation and balance. Strict vegetarians may be at more risk unless they are taking B_{12} supplements.

Overuse: No overuse effects are known; this vitamin is commonly prescribed as an energizer, for no known reason or proven effect.

Folic Acid

Sources: Dark-green vegetables, beef, wheat germ, dried beans, and peas have folic acid.

Function: Folic acid aids in the formation of red blood cells and genetic material.

Deficiency: A deficiency of folic acid causes anemia, smooth tongue, and diarrhea. Increased needs are noted in pregnancy and oral contraceptive use.

Overuse: No symptoms of overuse are known.

Pantothenic Acid

Sources: Pantothenic acid is found in plants, liver, kidney, whole grains, nuts, eggs, and dark-green vegetables. It is lost in refining and processing and is also manufactured by bacteria in the intestine.

Function: Pantothenic acid assists in the metabolism of carbohydrates, fats, and protein and in the formation of hormones and nerve-regulating substances.

Deficiency: Possible side effects of pantothenic acid deficiency are unknown.

Overuse: There are no known symptoms of too much pantothenic acid, although it will cause an increased need for thiamine.

Biotin

Sources: Egg yolk, liver, kidney, dark-green vegetables, and beans are sources of biotin. It is also manufactured by the bacteria in the intestine.

Function: Biotin aids in the formation of fatty acids and helps in the release of energy from carbohydrates.

Deficiency: No problems are associated with insufficient biotin.

Overuse: No symptoms of overuse are known.

Vitamin C—Ascorbic Acid

Sources: Citrus fruit, tomatoes, strawberries, melons, green peppers, potatoes, and dark-green vegetables contain vitamin C.

Function: Vitamin C aids in the formation of collagen, the structural fiber of the body and helps maintain the structure of the capillaries (the smallest blood vessels), teeth, and bones. Vitamin C is an antioxidant; i.e., it protects fats from oxidation and may prevent the formation of cancer-causing nitrosamines in the stomach from the ingestion of nitrates and nitrites.

Deficiency: Scurvy—characterized by bleeding gums, degenerated muscles, poor wound healing, loose teeth, and dry, rough skin—results from deficiencies of vitamin C.

Overuse: High dosage may cause withdrawal symptoms of scurvy when it is abruptly discontinued. Thus you need to taper the dosage slowly if you have been taking large doses. Pregnant women taking large doses of vitamin C can cause scurvy to occur in infants at birth. In addition, kidney stones, diarrhea, and an increased tendency to form blood clots have been noted.

Summary

In general, if you are eating a balanced diet with lots of complex carbohydrates and 6 ounces of low fat animal protein each day, there is no need to take any vitamin supplements. However, with all the processing and storage of food that occurs before it reaches your table, there may be significant vitamin loss.

Supplementation with a balanced multivitamin formula is probably harmless. We don't really know what good it does. We know how much to take to prevent vitamin deficiency, but we don't know how much to take for optimal health.

Megadosage of vitamins is unnecessary and potentially harmful.

In purchasing vitamins, get the cheapest brand that does not have artificial coloring added to it.

MINERALS: HOW MUCH IS TOO MUCH?

Minerals are organic substances that are not destroyed by cooking, food processing, or exposure to acid or air. Exposure to other substances in food may render minerals insoluble and unabsorbable.

Calcium

Calcium is the major constituent of bone and forms our infrastructure. It is our most prevalent mineral. A 160-pound person has 3 pounds of calcium, 98 percent of which is found in the bone, 1 percent in the tissues, and 1 percent in the teeth.

Sources: Milk and dairy products are the richest sources of calcium. It is also found in fish with soft bones, such as sardines, canned tuna, and canned salmon. Broccoli is also a rich source. (See Table 4-2). All we need is two glasses of skim milk or low-fat yogurt per day, and our daily calcium needs will be met (see discussion of osteoporosis in Chapter 1). The remainder of our calcium needs is supplied by vegetables and the other foods listed.

Function: In addition to being the cement that holds us upright, calcium has other vital functions. It helps control the flux of sodium and potassium across cell membranes, which is important in the ability of our muscles to contract and relax. It is also needed for the transmission of nerve impulses and for the functioning of enzyme systems. Bones are the reservoir, and there is a constant flux of calcium in and out of the bones, all influenced by specific hormones.

Calcium is a vitally important mineral. When our diet is deficient in it, the calcium needed will be drawn from the bones and teeth to support vital functions.

Deficiency: In children calcium deficiency will cause distorted bone growth (rickets), and in adults deficiency will cause thinning of the bones (osteoporosis).

Requirements: Men need 800 mg of calcium per day. Women who are premenopausal need 1000 mg per day; women who are postmenopausal need 1500 mg per day.

Absorption: Vitamin D is necessary for absorption. Dietary fat causes impaired absorption, and excess protein causes increased urinary calcium loss. Thus the traditional high fat, high protein, and low calcium diet in the United States can rapidly lead to calcium loss in the bones and to osteoporosis.

Overuse: Too much calcium may cause depression of nerve function, lethargy, drowsiness, ulcers, and calcium deposits in all the tissues of the body as well as kidney stones.

Table 4-2 shows the amount of calcium in various types of food.

Phosphorous

Phosphorous is a close working partner with calcium and is found in teeth and bones.

Sources: Meat, poultry, fish, milk, nuts, legumes, and cereals contain phosphorous.

Function: Phosphorous is a vital part of teeth and bones, is needed for the release of energy from carbohydrates and for the function of several B vitamins, and is used to transport fat around the body.

Deficiency: Prolonged use of antacids may cause phosphorous depletion.

Requirements: People need 80 mg of calcium per day. Pregnant women need more.

Overuse: No known problems are associated with too much phosphorous.

Sodium

The major source of sodium is table salt, which is sodium chloride. People have been using salt for all of recorded history. Orig-

Table 4-2 Calcium in Selected Foods

Food	Serving	Calcium (mg)
Dairy foods		
Cheese, cheddar	1 oz	150–250
Cheese, cottage	1 cup	150
Milk, nonfat dry	¼ cup	375
Milk, skim	8 oz	302
Milk, whole	8 oz	291
Yogurt, fruit	1 cup	345
Yogurt, plain	2 cups	415
Meats		
Oysters, raw	7–9	113
Salmon with bones	3 oz	300
Sardines with bones	3 oz	350
Tofu, processed with calcium sulfate	4 oz	150
Fruits and vegetables		
Beans, dried, cooked	1 cup	50–100
Broccoli	1 cup	36
Collards	½ cup	179
Kale	½ cup	103
Mustard greens	½ cup	97
Spinach	½ cup	100

inally, salt was used as a preservative for meat and fish, prior to the advent of refrigeration.

A certain amount of salt is needed, but we have extended our intake beyond what the body is capable of handling, resulting in water overload and high blood pressure.

Our ancestors consumed only the sodium that naturally occurred in the foods they ate, and in fact they ate one-quarter the amount of salt we do. Populations with low sodium diets hardly ever get high blood pressure, and their blood pressures never rise with age as they do in typical Western societies. The Japanese consume large amounts of salt and have high rates of blood pressure and strokes.

Our natural environment provides plenty of potassium and small amounts of sodium, and therefore our kidneys are designed to preserve sodium and excrete potassium. Excessive sodium consumption will cause excessive potassium excretion in the urine. This is why taking salt tablets to prevent dehydration can be dangerous. The potassium depletion may cause irregular heartbeats (arrhythmia) and sudden death. Don't take salt tablets, but drink fluids to prevent dehydration.

How Much Do We Eat?

We consume an average of 3 to 5 teaspoons of salt per day, which provides 7000 to 10,000 milligrams of sodium per day.

How Much Sodium Do We Need?

The body needs only ¼ teaspoon of salt per day. Safe consumption of sodium is about 1 teaspoon of salt per day (2300 mg of sodium). Since 1 gram of salt has 400 milligrams of sodium and 600 milligrams of chloride and there are 5.5 grams of salt in 1 teaspoon, we have our 2300 mg of sodium in one teaspoon.

Where Do We Find Sodium?

Approximately one-third of our sodium is found in the foods we eat, one-third is added at the table, and one-third is used in food preparation. We need to be aware of hidden sources of sodium such as many prepackaged, prepared, pickled, or processed foods. A large pickle has almost ½ teaspoon of salt. Look out for anything on a label that has sodium in it. Remember, it is the sodium that causes problems. Monosodium glutamate (MSG), sodium benzoate, sodium proprionate, sodium sulfate, disodium phosphate, sodium hydroxide, sodium caseinate, baking powder, and baking soda are all rich sources of sodium. Remember, too, that when you are reading a label, the ingredient found in the largest quantity is first, so if sodium is first or near the top of the label, there is too much. If it is at the end, it is probably in more acceptable quantities.

For further information see Table 4-3, which shows the sodium content of various foods.

How Do We Reduce Sodium Intake?

1. Do not add sodium at the table. Presalting food prior to eating will add about 1 teaspoon of salt before you have tasted it.

2. Limit your intake of foods that are naturally high in sodium or have a lot of sodium added to them (see table below).

3. Add only small amounts of salt to your food in food preparation, enough to keep the taste yet not enough to cause harm.

Salt is an acquired taste, and by reducing its intake, you can reeducate your taste buds to having less. After a few months you don't need the salt taste anymore; in fact, it will become less desirable.

We should learn to season our foods with small amounts of salt and other spices. If we cook a pot of soup that has 20 bowls of soup and we use 1 tablespoon (3 teaspoons) of salt for flavor, this is equal to about ⅐ teaspoon of salt in each bowl of soup. And ⅐ teaspoon of salt is 300 milligrams of sodium, which is not much.

Morton's Lite Salt is half sodium and half potassium. Therefore, it has only half the sodium content of regular salt. This is a good substitute for regular salt because of its reduced sodium content and the potassium it contains. However, you should be aware of some salt substitutes that are too high in potassium, as too much can be harmful.

Don't be afraid to use small amounts of salt; the food does not have to taste bland (see Table 4-3).

Table 4-3 The Sodium Content of Selected Foods

(We have listed only the foods with a high sodium content. All other foods generally have acceptable levels of sodium.)

Food	Protein Serving	Sodium (mg)
Cocoa mix	8 oz	232
Dairy products		
Cheese, American	1 oz	406
Cheese, blue	1 oz	396
Cheese, Camembert	1 oz	239
Cheese, cottage, regular	4 oz	457
Cheese, Edam	1 oz	274
Cheese, feta	1 oz	316
Cheese, Parmesan	1 oz	528
Milk, evaporated	1 cup	268–389
Milk, nonfat dry	½ cup	200–400
Fish and shellfish		
Crab	3 oz	314–425
Herring, smoked	3 oz	5234
Salmon, canned	3 oz	298–443
Sardines	3 oz	552
Shrimp, canned	3 oz	1955
Tuna	3 oz	288–303
Processed meats		
Bacon, Canadian	1 slice	394
Bacon, cooked	2 slices	274
Beef, canned	3 oz	802
Chicken frankfurter	1	714
Cold cuts	1 slice	200–300
Frankfurter or knockwurst	1	650

(*continued*)

Table 4-3   The Sodium Content of Selected Foods (*Continued*)

Food	Protein Serving	Sodium (mg)
Ham	3 oz	1114
Cereals		
Cheerios	1¼ cups	304
Corn Chex	1 cup	297
Total	1 cup	359
Wheaties	1 cup	355
Beans		
Baked	1 cup	606
Baked, with pork	1 cup	844
Kidney	1 cup	844
Nuts		
Cashews, dry roasted	1 cup	1200
Peanuts, salted	1 cup	600–900
Red	¼ cup	3708
White	¼ cup	2126
Soups, canned	1 cup	800–1200
Vegetables		
Asparagus, canned	1 cup	298
Beans	1 cup	900
Pickle, dill	1	928
Sauerkraut, canned	1 cup	1554
Miscellaneous		
Salt, onion, and garlic	1 tsp	1700–1900
Soy sauce	1 tbsp	1029
Teriyaki	1 tbsp	690

Source: *"The Sodium Content of Your Food,"* USDA Home and Garden Bulletin, no. 233, p. 198, revised 1983.

F I V E

Making Healthy Nutritional Choices

Eating the HealthMark way will show you that health food does not have to taste bland. We have over 100 restaurants in Denver that provide food prepared according to the HealthMark guidelines, and they have demonstrated that food definitely does not have to look brown and taste bland to be healthy. The recipes found in this book are also a testimony to this fact.

Together with the director of nutrition at HealthMark, Susan Stevens, and the many restaurants in Denver, we have been able to show that you can have food that looks and tastes the same as you are used to, only it is prepared differently. The success of the HealthMark program is due to two basic criteria: The food tastes good and is easy to prepare.

Before I get into specific recipes and examples of meal preparation, we need to discuss what to use and some alternatives to some of the "bad stuff."

THE UNDERLYING PRINCIPLES

The right choices—healthy choices—are all made under the following general principles:

1. Reduce the total fat intake to less than 45 grams of fat per day (1 tablespoon each of polyunsaturated and mono-unsaturated fats).

2. Keep the saturated fat intake as low as possible (less than 1 tablespoon per day).

3. Keep the polyunsaturated/saturated fat ratio at 2 to 1 or more.

4. Eat complex carbohydrates and reduce the sugar intake.

5. Eat 20 to 30 grams of fiber per day.

6. Have at least two glasses of skim milk or equivalent per day to provide the daily calcium needs, or take a calcium supplement.

7. Eat less than 2300 mg sodium per day, that is, 1 teaspoon of salt per day.

8. Keep your alcohol intake at a maximum of two drinks per day.

9. Reduce or eliminate both your consumption of artificial dyes and chemicals that may be cancer-causing as well as your intake of smoked foods.

10. *Eat three meals per day.*

COOKING METHODS

Do not fry your foods. The only people who can eat fried foods (provided that they are fried in good oils) are people who are at their ideal weight. Frying food adds unnecessary calories, and frying in polyunsaturated fat may lead to the formation of oxidized fats which may be cancer-causing substances. Always use fresh oil when frying, and don't do it often.

Food should be sautéed, poached, broiled, baked, and roasted. When roasting, always raise the food above the bottom of the roasting dish to allow excess fat to drain off; otherwise, the food cooks in the fat.

When sautéing food, use a nonstick pan and don't use butter. Use oils such as olive oil, canola oil, and other polyunsaturated oils, and use small quantities, e.g., a tablespoon instead of half a cup. If you do not want to use oil at all, you can sauté with a little broth or water in a nonstick pan.

Always remove the skin of chicken and turkey before cooking, and reduce cooking time to prevent drying out.

RED MEAT, POULTRY, AND FISH

The commonly eaten meats are no different from one another in fat and cholesterol content. Prime beef, pork, veal, and lamb all have 60 to 80 percent of their calories as fat.

In Colorado we are lucky to have a few sources of grass-fed natural beef that are not fed chemicals and hormones and are very lean. As I've said, these products are generally in the range of 23 to 30 percent of calories as fat and are as lean as chicken. These beef products can be eaten daily because of their low fat content.

The low fat beef products are more expensive, about the same price per pound as seafood. Buffalo and other wild game are even more lean and are great to eat, but watch out for game that is farm-grown specifically for slaughter and may be a lot more fatty than you want. Beefalo is generally lean, and in Colorado we have a source of lamb that is lean and clean.

Watch out for "lean beef products" in the supermarket, for example, the 88 percent lean ground beef. (See Table 3-5.) Buy your own round and grind it after it is zero-trimmed, or have the butcher grind it in front of you. Most store-bought ground beef has fat added to it. Always zero-trim any meat product before cooking, i.e., remove any visible fat.

Watch out for brands of beef labeled "organic" or "natural." They may indeed be organic or "natural" in that they are not fed hormones or antibiotics, and yet they are grown to be fat enough to be prime or choice beef. In the supermarket, "good" or "select" beef is generally as lean as the grass-fed natural beef; it is not guaranteed, however, to be free of hormones and antibiotics.

The leanest meats are from the hind quarter.

Cold cuts are filled with fat (70 to 80 percent of their calories), e.g., pastrami, corned beef, bologna, and other sausage. In addition, they generally contain red dye and nitrates that may be cancer-causing agents. Cold turkey cuts are the best to eat. Always try to find turkey prepared without nitrates.

The quantity of poultry (chicken and turkey) eaten in the United States is increasing, and unfortunately all that poultry may not be good. We are told to eat more chicken because it has much less fat than meats. This is true providing you skin the poultry before cooking. The fat is all in the skin, and without the skin it is lean. White meat is leaner than dark meat.

Unfortunately they feed the poultry the same "junk" as the cattle. Look for poultry that is not hormone- or antibiotic-fed, the so-called organic or free-range chickens. Many brands of "organic" poultry are available. Be sure to check them out before buying them.

Turkey franks and cold cuts made from turkey are not good because they may use good turkey meat but have added lots of fat and sodium to the products. Read the labels and calculate the fat content. Skinless, white poultry meat has about 20 percent and dark, skinless meat has about 30 to 35 percent of its calories as fat.

Duck and goose are too fatty to be eaten regularly and should be saved for an occasional treat. Pheasant is lean.

All fish contains the good fish fat that is polyunsaturated and assists in cholesterol and triglyceride lowering. Some fish contain more of the fat than others (see Table 3-7). However, we need to eat fish two to three times a week irrespective of whether it is fatty or not. This is not so much for the good fish oil—when you eat fish two to three times a week you are not eating high fat beef, and this reduces your intake of saturated fat and your risk of developing heart attacks.

Watch out for shrimp. Shrimp has a large amount of cholesterol and should be eaten sparingly. Even though shrimp have 260 to 300 mg of cholesterol in 6 ounces, they have only 10 percent fat, and this is the good fish fat. So there is a trade-off here. Shrimp, although not ideal, is always a better choice than high fat beef for "10 percent time."

DAIRY PRODUCTS

In terms of dairy products, 1 percent milk fat or preferably skim or nonfat products should be used. (Please refer to the Table 3-4 for a comparison of fat and cholesterol contents of these products.)

Cream, whole milk, 2 percent milk, half-and-half, and nondairy creamers (full of coconut oil) can always be replaced with nonfat milk, nonfat dry milk, evaporated nonfat milk, and equivalent yogurt or low fat cottage cheese products.

Nondairy creamers are filled with coconut oil and hydrogenated fats, which make them as bad or possibly worse than cream. Use skim milk or nonfat dry milk powder in your coffee or tea. (See the recipes in Appendix C for tips on making low fat sour cream, cream cheese, spreads, and low fat creamed soups.)

Butter and shortening should be avoided. Use good oils and soft margarine instead. Try to reduce the quantities used so that you do not affect the recipe. Experiment with your old recipes and have fun. When reducing the volumes of oil in a baking recipe, make up the liquid with skim milk.

Egg yolks should be avoided because of their very high cholesterol content. The fat in egg yolks is mostly saturated. (See Appendix C for egg white omelettes and scrambled egg whites.) When prepared well, most people cannot tell the difference between dishes prepared with egg whites and those prepared with egg yolks.

When baking, use two egg whites for each whole egg that the recipe calls for. If you were to use one whole egg in a cake and the other eggs as egg whites, using all whites might improve the texture, but experiment. The texture of your cakes may be fine without the yolk. One egg yolk in a whole cake will not add a large amount of cholesterol to each slice and is acceptable, provided that you do not eat the whole cake by yourself!

Cheese contains mostly saturated fat. (See Table 3-4.) Cream cheese is 95 percent fat, and hard cheeses are generally 75 percent fat. There is light cream cheese, e.g., Neufchatel or Philadelphia light which when calculated comes to 70 percent fat. These are too fatty to use.

The new hard cheeses made with part-skim milk, such as mozzarella, Romano, Jarlsberg, Ricotta, Parmesan, and Kraft light slices, are about 50 percent fat. These have too much fat to eat in large quantities but can be used in moderation.

A small amount of part-skim milk Parmesan cheese on your pasta does not add much fat, particularly if you are using a meatless sauce. One tablespoon of part-skim milk Parmesan or Romano cheese on your pasta will add 1 gram of fat. Therefore, even a few tablespoons are no real problem.

A pizza made with a thin crust and part-skim milk mozzarella cheese does not have much fat unless you order extra cheese or pepperoni or meatballs.

Ice cream was difficult to substitute until the development of low fat frozen yogurt, but buyer beware because all that is said to be low fat may not be. Most low fat frozen yogurts are 2 to 3 percent milk fat, which is too fat. Look for the low fat frozen yogurts that are 1 percent milk fat. There are some nonfat frozen yogurts as well. Some of these are so good that you cannot tell the difference between them and regular soft-serve ice cream. Remember, it may taste great and be low in fat, but it contains calories.

Italian ices and most sorbets are just sugar and water and have no fat, only calories.

Tofutti and Tofruzen are made with vegetable oils and do not have cholesterol. These foods contain large amounts of fat and therefore have plenty of calories.

HIGH CHOLESTEROL FOODS

There appears to be some contention that just eating foods high in cholesterol does not raise the blood cholesterol level. This is not so. Eating cholesterol will raise your blood cholesterol level. In addition we have already determined that eating saturated fat and cholesterol together raise your blood cholesterol very effectively. All foods that are high in cholesterol (organ meats and egg yolks) also contain saturated fats.

Shrimp are slightly different in that they are very high in cholesterol, and yet they are less than 10 percent fat, and the fat they contain is the good fish fat. There is a trade-off here. They can be eaten sparingly and never should be eaten in large quantities but mixed in with other seafood.

Saturated fat may be more potent in raising your blood cholesterol level than cholesterol itself, but high cholesterol-containing foods should still be avoided.

FATS AND OILS

When cooking and baking always use good fats (oils) rather than bad fats, and always try and use the *least amount of fat possible*.

Use olive oil or other polyunsaturated oils for sautéing. Canola oil (Puritan) is a good oil. It has mostly monounsaturated and some polyunsaturated fat and has the lowest saturated fat content of any oil fat. It has a good flavor. When a recipe calls for butter or shortening, use oil or margarine in smaller quantities, and always use the liquid or soft-tub varieties of margarine because they are the least saturated.

A good margarine should list liquid oil (either corn or safflower) as the first or second ingredient. In addition, it should have a P-S ratio of 2.5 to 1 or more.

Remember that adding unnecessary fat to your food adds unwanted calories. A teaspoon of margarine (or any fat) on your bread is an additional 45 calories, and a tablespoon of margarine (or any fat) on your corn is an extra 135 calories.

Avoid foods that are prepared with coconut and palm oils, such as crackers, breads, and baked goods. These oils are more saturated than butter. The crackers we eat are sometimes worse than the cheese placed upon them.

Mayonnaise is full of saturated fat and egg yolks and should be avoided. Some "lite" mayonnaise products are lower in fat (modified safflower oil) saturated fat, have more polyunsaturated fat, and do not contain cholesterol, but they still contain lots of fat (almost two-thirds of their calories). Most people will put 2 to 3 tablespoons on their sandwiches, a whopping amount of fat. Plain nonfat yogurt alone or mixed with a little Dijon mustard is a good topping for baked potatoes and is a mayonnaise substitute. (See Appendix C for a cole slaw dressing.) Lite safflower oil mayonnaise mixed with nonfat yogurt is an acceptable coleslaw dressing as well. (One-third lite mayonnaise plus two-thirds yogurt.)

PRESERVATIVES AND ADDITIVES

Chemicals are added to our food to enhance the color, flavor, and taste and to preserve their smell and shelf life. The average American consumes between 5 and 10 pounds of these chemicals each year, and this figure is rising. The use of artificial coloring rose from 3.7 million pounds in 1971 to 6.4 million pounds in 1984. These chemicals can cause anything from allergies to cancer, and should be avoided wherever possible.

Certain chemicals have been banned from use:

Dulcin in 1950 (artificial sweetener)

Safrole in 1960 (root beer flavoring)

Green no. 1 in 1966 (coloring)

Cobalt sulfate in 1966 (beer foam stabilizer)

Cyclamate in 1970 (artificial sweetener)

Violet no. 1 in 1973 (coloring)

Red no. 2 in 1976 (coloring)

Orange B in 1978 (coloring)

Let us look at the remainder of the chemicals by their function.

Preservatives

Preservatives are used to lengthen shelf life by inhibiting the growth of bacteria and fungi (molds) and to prevent the breakdown of fats causing them to become rancid. Salt was once used as a preservative for meat prior to the discovery of refrigeration.

BHT and BHA: BHT and BHA are among the most commonly used preservatives and are antioxidants; i.e., they retard the development of rancidity in oils and are used in potato chips, oils, cereals, and chewing gum. They have been implicated in cancer development in laboratory animals. Vitamins C and E are harmless antioxidants and can be used as substitutes for BHA and BHT—healthy choices.

Calcium (and sodium) propionate: Calcium and sodium propionate are considered safe and prevent bacterial and mold growth in baked goods.

EDTA: EDTA is a chelating agent used to remove metal contaminants in food. In large amounts it may inhibit the absorption of iron and calcium.

Propylgallate: Propylgallate is an antioxidant that occurs naturally in tea leaves. It is used to prevent fats from becoming rancid, has possibly been linked to the development of cancer, and is best avoided.

Sodium benzoate: Benzoic acid occurs naturally in fruit and this preservative is regarded as safe.

Sodium nitrate and sodium nitrite: Sodium nitrate and sodium nitrite are used as color and flavor enhancers as well as preservatives, in luncheon meats, smoked fish and meat, bacon, ham and frankfurters. Nitrites are broken down in the stomach into nitrosamines, which are potent cancer-causing agents.

Sorbic acid: This occurs naturally in berries of the mountain ash and is a safe replacement for nitrites.

Sulfiting agents: Sulfur dioxide, sodium bisulfite, and sodium sulfite are all used to retard bacterial growth and prevent discoloration of salads, wine, vegetables, and dried fruit. This food additive can cause severe allergic reactions and even death in susceptible people.

Emulsifiers

Emulsifiers enable water to mix with oil without separating. In salad dressing mustard is a good emulsifier.

Lecithin: Lecithin is an emulsifier and an antioxidant found mainly in egg yolks and soybeans. It is generally regarded as safe and is found in chocolate, ice cream, baked goods, and margarine. It does not lower blood cholesterol levels as is sometimes stated.

Monoglycerides and diglycerides: Monoglycerides and diglycerides are regarded as safe emulsifiers and are generally found in highly refined foods.

Polysorbates 60, 65, and 80: These are regarded as safe emulsifiers.

Brominated vegetable oil (BVO): Brominated vegetable oil (BVO) is stored in the body fat and is cause for concern. Safer emulsifiers are available.

Thickeners and Stabilizers

These are used to improve the consistency and texture of food.

Carboxymethylcellulose: Cellulose gum is used in diet preparations because it retains water and keeps you feeling full. It is also used in ice cream, jelly, and beer.

Gums: Guar, locust bean, arabic, furcelleran, ghatti, karaya, and tragacanth are all thickeners. They are used to stabilize beer foam (arabic) and to prevent sugar crystals from forming in candy, ice cream, and desserts. In small amounts they are regarded as safe.

Carrageenan: Obtained from seaweed, carrageenan is probably safe in small amounts.

Modified starches: Modified starches are safe and are used in soups and gravies as thickening agents.

Sodium alginate: Sodium alginate is regarded as safe in small amounts.

Sodium caseinate: Sodium caseinate is derived from the protein in milk and is safe.

Flavor Enhancers

Disodium guanylate: Disodium guanylate is found in certain mushrooms and fish. The body converts it into uric acid, which can cause gout attacks and kidney stones.

Monosodium glutamate: Monosodium glutamate (MSG) is used in many foods and is believed to cause the "Chinese restaurant syndrome" (burning sensation in the back of the neck and forearms, tightness in the chest, and headache) in some adults.

Hydrolyzed vegetable protein: Hydrolyzed vegetable protein (HVP) is safe to use as a flavor enhancer.

Artificial Colorings

These colorings are usually used in junk food and thus should be avoided. Most are associated with allergic types of reactions, and some may be linked to cancer.

The dyes that are generally considered as safe in that they are usually only associated with allergic reactions are yellow dyes nos. 5 and 6. Red dye no. 40 is the most widely used dye, and tests on its safety are inconclusive.

In general, it is best to avoid artificial dyes whenever possible.

Why expose yourself to a possible danger when safer alternatives are available? Carotene and other natural coloring agents are a better alternative.

LABEL READING

If we are truly what we eat, the ingredient lists on many labels should give us cause to think. How many of the ingredients that you ate today can you identify?

We should always look for the freshest and least processed foods available and become regular label readers. Our consumption of packaged foods has risen to about 55 percent of everything we eat. By law labels are not allowed to lie, but they are often confusing and misleading. The following guidelines should help you read labels more effectively.

Ingredient List

The first ingredient listed is the one that is contained in the greatest amount, i.e., there is more of that item than any other in the product. The information you do not receive is the exact amount of each item listed, and so you have to make value judgments based on what foods or additives you are trying to avoid.

1. *Fats* are very rarely listed as saturated or unsaturated. If you see animal fat, lard, beef tallow, milk, butter fat, hydrogenated or partially hydrogenated vegetable oil, coconut oil, palm oil, or cocoa butter on a label, the product contains saturated fats.

    Beware of the label that says that this product may contain "one or more of the following vegetable oils" and may include a list of unsaturated oils as well as palm oil, coconut oil, or a hydrogenated oil. It is best to avoid this product as it is impossible to tell which oil has been used.

2. *Sugars* are frequently hidden throughout the label and need to be picked out. Sugar is often listed under a va-

riety of names and forms to hide the fact that so much is present. Any word ending in *-ose* is sugar: maltose, dextrose, sucrose, fructose, lactose, and galactose. Beware the so-called natural sugars. There is no such thing: All sugar is natural. Brown sugar is sugar with molasses, molasses is sugar, as are honey, corn syrup, maple syrup, and corn syrup solids.

3. *Salt* is generally considered to be table salt, which is sodium chloride. It is the sodium that is associated with all the health problems, and thus you need to read labels looking for anything with sodium, e.g., monosodium glutamate and sodium benzoate. Some products are switching to potassium instead of sodium, such as potassium benzoate, which has replaced sodium benzoate in diet soda and has helped reduce the sodium content.

Nutrition Labels

Many products provide nutrition labels, and I hope all products will be required to do so in the future. Look for the following:

Serving Size

Don't make the mistake of thinking that the stated serving size is the whole package. If you are watching your caloric intake, this is the easiest way to be misled. Many products such as high calorie granolas will tell you that each serving is only 140 calories; however, what you usually miss is that each serving is only one-quarter of a cup. Not many people will eat one-quarter of a cup of granola for breakfast. They will eat at least one cup, which is 560 calories, without the milk.

Calories

Calories refer to the number of calories per serving (see the example in "Serving Size.") Many low calorie foods will mislead you in this way by listing a small serving size and a small number of calories. Reduced calorie labels must be at least one-third less calories per serving than the regular equivalent.

Protein

Protein is usually stated in the number of grams of protein present and says nothing about the quality of the protein.

Carbohydrate

Many products do not differentiate between simple (sugars) and complex carbohydrates (starches), although most cereals are doing this now.

Fats

Most products, except for margarines, do not label the fat as saturated or unsaturated. When this information is available, you can calculate the P-S ratio, which should be 2.5 or more.

You should keep the percentage of calories as fat in a particular food item at less than 20 to 25 percent.

The number of grams of fat present are important as you need to keep within the guidelines already set, that is, 45 grams total and 15 grams each of the monounsaturated and polyunsaturated fats and less than 15 grams of saturated fat.

Remember that 1 teaspoon of fat is the same as one "pat" of fat (butter or margarine) and contains 5 grams of fat. One tablespoon of fat is 15 grams of fat. A teaspoon and a tablespoon have 45 and 135 calories in them, respectively.

Percentage of the RDA

The recommended daily allowance (RDA) is listed for 19 nutrients and is the amount of these nutrients needed daily to prevent deficiencies. These percentages are listed without regard for specific age and sex or special needs. Manufacturers do not need to list all 19 nutrients, and generally only those that contain 2 percent or more of the RDA are listed.

Other Items

Enriched and *fortified* are often found on labels. Enrichment often refers to the replacement of vitamins and minerals lost in the refining process of grains and cereals. This process does not replace all the nutrients lost and never replaces the fiber removed. Beware of breads that are brown in color and are labeled to contain wheat flour. All flour is from wheat, and it is not whole wheat unless so stated. These breads are usually white flour with a coloring to make them look like whole wheat.

"Fortified" refers to the addition of nutrients not normally found in the food. Milk is fortified with vitamin D, which helps with the absorption of the calcium from milk.

Other items of interest are "organic" or "natural" labels. At a national level these have no legal definition, and some states are trying to regulate this. *Organic* usually refers to a product that is grown without the use of fertilizers, pesticides, and additives. *Natural* should but may not mean that nothing artificial is added to the product. Read the labels.

EATING OUT

Dining out is social, pleasurable, and a necessity for some people who just don't cook. We are a society that eats out a lot, and we have to learn to manage our new lifestyle in this situation.

In Denver this really is not much of a problem. We have over 100 restaurants that have HealthMark-approved items on their menus. In fact, these are so popular that some restaurants sell 30 to 40 percent of all items on the menu as HealthMark selections. This has enabled the graduates of HealthMark programs to eat out easily, without having to worry about whether the restaurant will or won't make the food properly. It also saves some people the embarrassment of having to order special food. This is a program that is unique in its success. We have every type of restaurant on our list from diners to the fanciest restaurants in Denver.

Many restaurants all over the United States already have Health-Mark-approved items on their menus and are not even aware of it. Always ask how the food is prepared. Often the new light cuisine type of foods are okay. They are using good oils instead of butter, for example.

There are very few restaurants in which you cannot eat. They can always modify something on the menu to comply with your new eating habits. If they are not prepared to do so, then go somewhere else. Remember, you pay for the service, and if they are not prepared to accommodate you, leave.

Breakfast

Breakfast is usually not too difficult. The hardest part used to be getting skim milk for your cereal, but that is becoming less of a hassle. High fiber cereals are always available, and good old oatmeal is still the best. Make sure it is not instant oatmeal (less fiber, with salt and fat added). If no skim milk is available dilute the regular milk with water (⅓ cup milk to ⅔ cup water) or use apple juice.

Toast should always be wheat toast, dry, that is, without butter. If you don't ask, it will automatically be served with butter on it.

You can always ask them to make an egg white omelette, although this is sometimes a culture shock for chefs. It is fun to order it and watch their reaction.

Lunch

For most of us dinner is our main meal, and thus we should eat a lighter lunch. It makes more sense to eat lunch as the main meal so that we don't consume excess calories at night, but this is usually not socially possible. If you can do this, swap the lunch and dinner suggestions.

Save your animal protein for your main meal. Therefore, lunch should be light: soups and salads, pasta dishes, fruit plates, or, if you are brown-bagging it, yogurt, bagels or bread, rolls, and fruit.

For salad dressings always ask for the dressing on the side and use the vinaigrette dressing or ask for oil and vinegar and make your own, or just use lemon juice or balsamic vinegar, a wonderfully flavored vinegar that makes a great salad dressing by itself.

If egg is served in the salad, eat the white and not the yolk. Don't eat the ham, and if chicken or tuna is in the salad, make sure it's not large amounts: 1 to 2 ounces is fine.

If eating a turkey sandwich, don't eat it deli-style with 4 to 6 ounces of turkey but get it with 1 to 2 ounces of turkey. Use mustard instead of mayonnaise on the bread or use a lite safflower oil mayonnaise in small quantities. A tuna sandwich or a chicken salad sandwich is usually made with regular mayonnaise. (The lite mayonnaise and yogurt mix is also good for tuna and chicken salad sandwiches.)

When eating pasta, ask whether the noodle is made with eggs. Most restaurant noodles are. Most store-bought "Italian" noodles are not made with eggs unless egg noodle is specified on the box. One cup of cooked noodles made with eggs has 50 mg of cholesterol. If this is to be your cholesterol-free meal, 50 to 150 mg of cholesterol is going to add up quickly.

It is hard to find egg-free noodles in restaurants, which makes eating pasta difficult. However, if you are eating pasta as the main meal of the day (when you are supposed to eat the animal protein) and it does not have lots of animal protein (meat) in the sauce, then the amount of cholesterol you are getting is of no real consequence.

Dinner

Dinner is your main meal and where you would expect to eat your 6 ounces of animal protein. Obviously, when eating red meats (beef, veal, lamb, and pork) in restaurants, you are going to get the fattiest, choice cuts. They should be avoided. We have some restaurants in Denver that use our low fat beef for hamburgers, steaks, and stir-fries, but this is the exception.

Eat chicken and fish, and leave out the sauces or have them served on the side. Always ask how the chicken or fish is broiled, baked, or poached. Tell them to use a little oil to prevent sticking to cooking surfaces, but to avoid using butter, even what is called "light butter." There is no such thing. Light sauces are usually filled with fat—ask what's in them.

Appetizers can be noncreamed soups or salads. The entrée should be served with steamed vegetables; however, the vegetable should not be steamed in butter—a small amount of oil can be used.

Desserts should be fresh fruit or used for 10 percent time. Angel food cake made with egg whites is a great base for "legal" dessert.

Friends' Houses and Social Functions

There are times to be polite and tell friends that you have certain dietary requirements without intimidating them, and then there are times when you have to bite the bullet.

I have the philosophy that if someone gives me a cigarette, I don't have to smoke it to be polite. If you are faced with a situation that you cannot control, you have a variety of options:

1. Eat before you go so that you are not hungry and can nibble without being impolite.

2. Eat what you can and nibble at the remainder. If there is a lardaceous piece of prime rib staring up at you from the plate, you can eat 3 ounces of it and thus limit the amount of saturated fat and cholesterol eaten. Eat the vegetables, rice, and potatoes. They will probably have small amounts of butter which may be insignificant, but remember this all adds up. Eat the bread and salad, watching out for the dressing.

3. You can write it off as 10 percent time and eat without a guilty conscience, providing you return to 90 percent time the next day.

I will usually try the first or second choices and will never go hog-wild, because extremely fatty foods make me ill. I will pick my way around what I can and can't eat and usually wait for dessert.

When I do go wild, it's usually at a time of my choosing and with foods of my choice. I always feel that it is better psychologically to do it when you are in control. It is always better to be in control when you are "junking out" so that you are in control of your eating habits.

At organized functions or banquets with preset meals, get in the habit of calling up and inquiring what is being served. If it is the "prime rib dinner," ask for chicken, salmon, or a fruit plate. If this is not available, then eat before you go. If they serve salmon or chicken baked in sauce, then push the sauce to the side to minimize the fat intake.

On airplanes preorder the food. You need to give a 24-hour advance notice. The biggest problem is not just the food but also getting what you ordered. Mostly it is just not delivered, so you are stuck with what is served. Usually it is chicken, and you can get by. If not, then do what is needed to survive.

On airplanes you cannot order more than one choice, so in my experience ordering low cholesterol meals is the safest. The food is usually edible and conforms with our dietary guidelines for the most part. No one ever said airplane food was supposed to be good.

ALCOHOL

The greatest danger in alcohol use and abuse is denial. Alcohol is a drug that is used socially, and its occasional use does no harm. Prolonged or chronic use can lead to addiction and all the associated medical problems: liver damage and cirrhosis, for example, and ulcers, nutritional deficiencies, high blood pressure, and cardiac, nerve, and brain damage.

There is some evidence that two drinks a day will elevate your HDLs and possibly protect you from developing heart attacks. This is a dangerous statement, and no one should recommend two drinks a day to anyone as therapy because of the inherent dangers of chronic alcohol use and abuse. You can raise your HDLs by exercising, and in fact you raise the good type of HDL with exercise (see pages 47–48).

Remember that each drink you take has the same alcohol content and therefore the same number of calories. One shot of hard liquor (1.5 ounces), a 5-ounce glass of wine, and a 12-ounce bottle of beer all have about 150 calories. There is no difference in their alcohol content, and therefore there is no difference between hard and soft liquor. It is a social distinction. These are empty calories and are usually taken with other high calorie foods, e.g., potato chips and nuts, which go a long way to promote the development of obesity.

A few drinks every now and then are of no real consequence as long as you don't drink and drive. If you drink every day, ask yourself why. You may have a problem.

FAST FOODS

There is nothing redeeming about fast food. The whole concept is misguided and goes against every basic nutritional principle. All fast foods supply you with very high calorie foods that are basically empty calories (sugar and fat). The foods lack fiber and vitamins and are loaded with sugar, salt, fat, and cholesterol.

Don't be fooled into eating the fish or chicken, because they are deep-fried in beef tallow (fat) or lard (pork fat). Each little chicken nugget has 1 teaspoon of fat (mostly saturated) and turns out to be worse than eating some of the hamburgers. Some fast-food chains now advertise that they use vegetable oils to fry their food, but they are using hydrogenated oils or shortening. Beware! See Table 5-1 for a listing of the fat and salt content of some fast foods.

You can get salads at some of the fast-food chains. Make sure that they are not treated with sulfiting agents because of possible allergies, and watch out for the dressings. Don't take the kids there to eat hamburgers while you eat the salad; the whole family should eat the salad. Baked potatoes are available at some of the chains. Watch out for the toppings; they are full of fat.

Table 5-1   Fat and Salt Content of Selected Fast Foods

	Calories	Fat (g)	Percentage of Calories Consumed as Fat	Sodium (mg)
Arby's				
Junior roast beef sandwich	220	9	37	530
Roast beef deluxe sandwich	486	23	42	1298
French fries	216	12	50	39
Vanilla shake	330	11	30	275
Burger King				
Hamburger	310	12	35	560
Cheeseburger	360	16	40	705
Whopper	670	38	51	975
Double Beef Whopper	890	53	54	1015
Double Beef Whopper with cheese	980	61	56	1295
Chicken sandwich	690	42	55	775
French fries	210	11	47	230
Chocolate shake	340	10	26	280
Domino Pizza				
Cheese, 12-inch, 2 slices	340	6	16	660
Pepperoni, 12-inch, 2 slices	380	12	28	880
Kentucky Fried Chicken				
Drumstick	117	7	54	207
Side breast	199	12	54	558
Thigh	257	18	63	566

(continued)

Table 5-1   Fat and Salt Content of Selected Fast Foods
(*Continued*)

	Calories	Fat (g)	Percentage of Calories Consumed as Fat	Sodium (mg)
Side breast, extra crispy	286	18	57	564
Thigh, extra crispy	343	23	60	549
McDonalds				
Hamburger	263	11	38	506
Quarter Pounder	427	24	50	718
Quarter Pounder with cheese	525	32	55	1220
Big Mac	570	35	55	979
Filet-O-Fish	435	26	54	799
Chicken McNuggets, 6 pieces	323	21	59	512
French fries	220	12	49	109
Egg McMuffin	340	16	42	885
Sausage McMuffin with egg	517	33	57	1044
Vanilla shake	352	8	20	201
Pizza Hut				
Thin 'N Crispy pizza				
Beef, 10-inch, 3 slices	490	19	35	N/A
Cheese, 10-inch, 3 slices	450	15	30	N/A
Pepperoni, 10-inch, 3 slices	430	17	36	N/A
Thick 'N Chewy pizza				
Beef, 3 slices, 10-inch	620	20	29	N/A

(*continued*)

Table 5-1   Fat and Salt Content of Selected Fast Foods
(*Continued*)

	Calories	Fat (g)	Percentage of Calories Consumed as Fat	Sodium (mg)
Cheese, 3 slices, 10-inch	560	14	22	N/A
Pepperoni, 3 slices, 10-inch	560	18	29	N/A
Taco Bell				
Bean burrito	343	12	31	272
Beef burrito	466	21	40	327
Burrito Supreme	457	22	43	367
Taco	186	8	39	79
Wendy's				
Hamburger, single	350	18	46	410
Hamburger, double	560	34	87	575
Hamburger, double with cheese	630	40	57	835
Chicken sandwich	320	10	28	500
French fries	280	14	45	95
Bacon and cheese baked potato	570	30	47	1180
Cheese baked potato	590	34	53	450
Sour cream and chives baked potato	460	24	47	230

Note: Remember that 5 grams of fat equal 1 teaspoon and 15 grams of fat equal 1 tablespoon. Calculate how many teaspoons or tablespoons of fat are in the above items. A Double Beef Whopper with cheese, fries, and a vanilla shake have 83 grams of fat, which is 5½ tablespoons of fat. There are also 1825 calories in this snack.

Source: M. J. Franz, *Fast Food Facts*, International Diabetes Center, Park Nicollet Medical Foundation, 1984, revised 1985.

SIX

Getting the Most Out of Exercise

PUTTING EXERCISE BACK INTO OUR LIVES

Exercise has specific physical and psychological benefits and plays an important role in the development of an effective lifestyle change.

Before the age of mechanization and mechanical transportation, we were much more physically active in our jobs and lifestyles. Today we have automobiles, trains, planes, and buses to get us around, and we also have televisions that keep us from enjoying physical activity.

Our children are becoming less and less fit and more and more obese and unhealthy. The fitness craze that appears to be affecting a portion of the adult population seems to be bypassing our children, and this is a tragedy in the making.

Because we have lost all this natural physical activity that was a normal part of our daily lives, we need to build in exercise time as part of our daily routine.

The Physical Benefits of Exercise

1. Exercise lowers your blood pressure. The immediate effect of exercise is to raise the systolic blood pressure, but the prolonged effect is to cause a relaxation and dilata-

tion of the arteries, thus lowering the blood pressure. In addition, exercise causes the release of naturally tranquilizing hormones—endorphins—which reduce stress levels and lower blood pressure.

2. Exercise aids in weight loss by burning calories. No weight-loss program will be effective or sustained unless exercise is an integral part of the program. (See Table 8-2 for calories burned with exercise.)

3. Exercise, especially weight-bearing exercise, makes strong bones by retaining calcium in the bones, thus preventing osteoporosis.

4. Exercise will protect you from heart disease by elevating your HDL levels. It also will reduce the tendency for the blood to form clots, making the risk of heart attack and stroke less likely. Chronic exercise will also dilate (widen) your coronary arteries and strengthen the heart muscle.

5. Exercise increases lung capacity.

6. Exercise stimulates the large intestine and helps to regulate bowel movements.

The Psychological Benefits of Exercise

1. Endorphins are released. These morphinelike, naturally tranquilizing hormones released by the brain give rise to the euphoria after exercise, the "runners' high." Because of this, exercise is regarded as the best physiological tranquilizer and helps reduce anxiety symptoms (but not the causes). Endorphins are released after about 30 minutes of aerobic exercise.

2. There is a feeling of achievement with exercise that helps to boost your self-esteem. This together with the endor-

phin effect will be helpful in treating depression. There is no substitute for looking and feeling great.

3. Exercise also will improve your sleep patterns, your ability to concentrate, and your sex life.

I like to do my exercise at noon because of the stress-relieving effects. It gives me something to look forward to in the morning and helps me sail through the rest of the afternoon. This enables me physically and emotionally to handle the long and sometimes exhausting hours I work. There is nothing wrong with working long and hard hours, if you keep yourself in great shape, physically and emotionally.

Some people like to exercise in the evening and others in the morning. It does not matter when you exercise, only that you do it.

What Form of Exercise Should You Do?

There are many forms of exercise, but the important changes listed above will only be experienced with what is called *aerobic exercise*.

Aerobic Exercise

Aerobic exercise places such demands on the body that it is required to improve its ability to handle oxygen. It involves large muscle groups, needs to be maintained continuously, and is rhythmical in nature. Examples are running, jogging, walking, hiking, swimming, skating, bicycling, rowing, cross-country skiing, rope skipping, and various endurance games.

Aerobic exercise is done within the body's need to utilize and transport oxygen and is by definition endurance, working at 60 to 85 percent of your maximal heart rate.

Anaerobic Exercise

Anaerobic exercise is done without the need for oxygen and thus cannot be sustained for long periods. Sprinting is an example.

Anaerobic exercise has no benefits other than for speed training and for increasing levels of fitness such as in interval training. Interval training involves repeated short, fast bursts of exercise with a short recovery in between to allow the muscles to improve their ability to utilize oxygen. Anaerobic exercise does nothing for protection from heart attacks.

Isometric Exercises

Isometric exercise involves the chronic, sustained contraction of muscles and is designed to increase muscle mass rather than cardiovascular fitness. Isometric exercise can elevate blood pressure and is dangerous for people with high blood pressure.

Isotonic Exercise

Weight lifting and calisthenics are examples of isotonic exercises. Again, this builds muscle strength and bulk and does not improve cardiovascular fitness. Many bodybuilders have great bodies and yet are poorly conditioned and get no cardiovascular protection from their exercise. Isotonics can also elevate blood pressure.

Circuit and supercircuit training are becoming popular in health clubs across the United States. They combine weight lifting and aerobic conditioning and produce cardiovascular fitness.

How Do You Measure a Good Workout?

To assess whether you are getting an adequate aerobic workout, you must know what your training heart rate should be.

At HealthMark we use 60 to 85 percent of your maximal heart rate. Your maximal heart rate is defined as 220 beats per minute minus your age, or the maximal heart rate achieved with a maximal treadmill stress test. If you are 40 years old, for example, then your maximal heart rate is 220 minus 40 or 180 beats per minute. Your training heart rate should be 60 to 85 percent of this, which is 108 to 153 beats per minute.

The most specific way to measure your maximal and training heart rates is to have a maximal treadmill stress test. This test gives us a very specific way to assess how fit you are and how your heart and blood pressure respond to the challenge of exercise.

No one with any major risk factors for heart disease or over the age of 35 should begin an exercise program without a maximal treadmill stress test. Good exercise is safe exercise.

Developing an Adequate Exercise Program

There are a number of factors to consider in developing an adequate exercise program. These are the guidelines we use at HealthMark.

1. *Frequency:* Four to six days a week. It is always good to take off 1 day a week. Some people are advised to exercise 7 days a week, e.g., diabetics who want to maintain a consistent control over their blood sugar levels and people with obesity and high blood pressure who want to achieve faster results. Three days is the barest minimum and is a maintenance level rather than a level used to achieve fitness.

2. *Intensity:* Your heart rate (pulse) should be kept within the training rate determined by your stress test or calculated as above. Your pulse should be checked every 10 to 15 minutes by stopping exercise and counting your pulse for 15 seconds and multiplying by 4. If your pulse rate is too low then increase the intensity, and if it is too high reduce the intensity of the exercise.

3. *Duration:* Thirty-five to sixty minutes of exercise should be done. Duration and intensity are dependent on each other—the lower the intensity the longer the duration, and vice versa. Total fitness in the nonathletic adult is best achieved by low- to moderate-intensity activity carried out for longer periods.

4. *Mode of activity:* It does not matter what you do as long as it is aerobic in nature as defined above. Varying the type of activity may help with compliance.

How Much is Enough?

Recent studies have shown that to protect yourself from heart disease you need to burn about 2000 calories per week. This is equivalent to 18 to 20 miles of fast walking or jogging per week. This approximates 35 to 45 minutes of aerobic activity at least four to five times per week, and you will never achieve this goal with the old recommendations of 25 minutes three times per week (unless you can run 5-minute miles).

Beyond this there is no added cardiovascular protection, and the HDL levels do not increase any more. When you exceed these levels of exercise, you are exercising for something other than cardiovascular protection, e.g., for improved fitness, for training for marathons and triathalons, for stress relief, and in some cases for pure enjoyment. Three times a week is the barest maintenance level when fitness is achieved.

WHAT ARE THE HEALTHMARK GUIDELINES?

Once you have determined your training heart rate and have learned how to take your pulse your exercise program can be built as follows: Always begin with a 5-minute warm-up and end with a 5-minute cool down (see below). The aerobic phase should initially be 30 to 35 minutes for the first 1 to 2 weeks. Don't be afraid to try to exercise for this length of time. Most people can achieve this with ease and will have to restrain themselves from doing more. The urge to overdo exercise is great when you first start. However, some of you may not be able to make the 30 minutes and may have to stop intermittently until you are able to make it without stopping. Keep on doing it until you reach this level.

Once you are comfortable at this level (after 1 to 2 weeks) you move up to 40 to 50 minutes per session, this should last a week or two. Then you can move up to 45 to 60 minutes per session. You should always do one longer slower exercise session per week on weekends, e.g., in the first phase a 40- to 45- minute session on Saturdays; in phase two, a 50- to 55-minute session; and in phase three, up to 60 minutes or longer.

If you want to jog, begin with a walk-jog program and you can build the jogging up steadily by walking less and jogging more as you get fitter and stronger. Beginning jogging immediately will cause too much stress on your joints and will result in injuries. Be patient and go slow.

Some of you will have trouble getting your heart rates up to the prescribed level with walking outdoors and may need to jog. This is why the treadmill is such a great exercise tool. Walking is comfortable up to a level of 4 miles per hour, and after this you need to begin to jog. However, on a treadmill you can slow the speed down and elevate it in order to increase the workload and get your heart rate up.

It does not matter what you do, only that you get your heart rate up to the prescribed level.

Exercising more frequently in the beginning will help you achieve your goals quicker; once you are at your ideal weight and have no risk factors, the maintenance level of burning 2000 calories per week can be maintained. At HealthMark we also work on the principle of hard and easy days to add some variety. Hard days can be defined as either working at a higher heart rate (intensity) or by working for a longer time (duration) and vica versa for slower days.

A Typical HealthMark Week

Monday—easy day—35 to 50 minutes at lower-end heart rate

Tuesday—hard day—35 to 50 minutes at high-end heart rate

Wednesday—easy day—35 to 50 minutes at lower-end heart rate

Thursday—hard day—35 to 50 minutes at high-end heart rate

Friday—easy day—35 to 50 minutes at lower-end heart rate

Saturday—hard day—45 to 60 minutes at high-end heart rate

Sunday—rest day

Each session is preceded by a warm-up and should end with a cool-down.

Warm-up

Exercise begun without adequate warm-up can induce electro-cardiographic abnormalities which can be dangerous, particularly for people with heart disease. Inadequate warm-up can also lead to injuries such as muscle pulls, strains, and lower back problems. The gradual increase in heart rate will assist the heart in preparation for the increased blood flow associated with exercise. All bodily systems must be prepared for the increased stresses demanded by exercise.

Care should be taken to warm up adequately, especially if it is cold or damp, and a longer warm-up should be taken if you feel stiff and inflexible. People with heart disease, high blood pressure, and vascular disease of the legs should warm up for at least 7 to 10 minutes.

The warm-up session should begin with 5 minutes (or more if indicated) of slow walking, light jogging, or cycling. This should be followed by a few minutes of light stretching, e.g., ankle twirls, shoulder rotations, and light calf, hamstring, and quadriceps stretches. Light stretching should be done prior to exercise because the muscles are stiff. More serious stretching can be done after the exercise session when the muscles are fully warmed up.

If you like to exercise first thing in the morning, you should take care to spend more time with easy stretching and warm-up because your muscles are very stiff after a night of sleep.

Cool-down

An equally important part of your exercise program is to cool down. After exercise blood can pool in the legs, and if light activity is not continued, dizziness and even fainting can occur because of inadequate blood flow to the brain.

Light activity continued after the workout allows the muscles to squeeze the blood back to the heart and prevents pooling in the legs. This should be done for 5 minutes and be followed by stretching to prevent muscle soreness. (See suggested stretches, page 189.) Pooling of blood and the resultant low blood pressure can be dangerous for people with heart disease.

After the workout a warm but not hot shower should be taken. Hot showers can induce dilatation of the blood vessels, which will also cause pooling of blood and the above-listed complications, especially for cardiac patients.

How Many Calories Do We Burn with Exercise?

The number of calories burned with exercise depend on the type, the duration, and the intensity of the particular activity. Table 8-2 gives ranges for calories burned in a variety of different exercises. The number of calories also depends on the height and weight of the individual. The heavier and taller you are, the more calories you burn for a similar activity. In addition, being at a higher altitude will also burn a few extra calories because the air has less oxygen.

One bowl of peanuts is 800 calories and is equivalent to 6 to 7 miles of fast walking or jogging. If this is consumed with a couple of drinks at 150 calories each, you have eaten 1100 calories as a snack. This represents 9 to 10 miles of running or 14 to 16 miles of walking. A doughnut is about 400 calories, or 3.5 miles of running. A piece of apple pie (600 calories) is 5 miles of running.

Clothing

Clothing should be loose fitting and comfortable and should be adapted to the environmental conditions. Loose-fitting clothes prevent chafing and allow for unobstructed movement, whereas tight-fitting clothing may restrict blood flow to the working muscles. Clothes should be in bright colors or with reflective material to increase visibility.

Proper shoes should be worn for the specific event. The best shoe is not the most expensive but the one that fits best and is best suited for a particular activity. A running shoe is no good for racket sports or aerobics and will cause injury; likewise, racket and aerobics shoes are not good for running.

Pay special attention to the wear on your shoes. It is always better to replace them if they are showing signs of wear. Running shoes lose their cushioning, and the heel counters break down fairly soon. A good rule of thumb is to change the shoes when you begin to develop any aches or pains in the legs or feet.

Exercising in the Heat

The body temperature rises with exercise, and it is vital to get rid of this heat. We do this by evaporating sweat (our air conditioning). This is easily affected by humidity, clothing, and internal fluid levels. Hot, humid days present the greatest danger. When the humidity rises, the moisture content of the air is high, and you cannot evaporate fluids to cool down (you only sweat). This is also the case if you are wearing clothing that covers too much of your body or are dehydrated: You cannot evaporate fluids and cool down.

To prevent heat injuries such as heat stroke or heat exhaustion, you should adhere to the following guidelines:

1. Avoid exercising in extreme heat and high humidity. Try to exercise indoors in an air-conditioned facility or exercise in the early morning or evening when it is cooler.

2. If you do exercise outdoors, reduce the intensity and duration of the activity.

3. Be able to recognize the warning signs of heat injury.

4. Increase fluid intake prior to, during, and after exercise.

5. Wear loose-fitting, cotton clothing to assist in evaporation. Leave your extremities exposed to aid in evaporation.

6. Shade the head and neck by wearing the appropriate headgear.

7. Exercise in the shade when possible to avoid constant exposure to the sun's harmful rays. Wear at least a number 15 or higher sun block that does not wash off with sweating.

8. Acclimatization to the heat will usually take 7 to 14 days.

Exercising in the Cold

Cold weather presents fewer problems than the heat. Exercise will generate additional body heat that is used to maintain normal temperature. The hands, feet, and head represent the greatest risk from the cold and need to be protected. The natural tendency of the body is to restrict blood flow to the extremities to maintain a normal body core temperature in cold weather.

Wind and higher air moisture increase the effects of the cold. Wet clothing, caused by rain or sweating, will lose its insulating ability and may magnify the effects of the cold. Wear clothing made from polypropylene that does not retain moisture and that wicks moisture away from the skin. The outer layers of clothing should be made from a waterproof and windproof fabric, such as Gore-Tex. It is most important to dress in layers and to keep the hands and head covered.

Snow-covered and icy surfaces require greater energy expenditure to maintain balance and increase the likelihood of injury due to unexpected falls and slips. Shoes should have good tread and traction.

To exercise safely in the cold, you should follow these guidelines:

1. Allow extra time for warm-up.

2. Stay close to home so that you can get home easily if you get cold or the weather changes for the worse.

3. Try to avoid head winds that will increase the windchill.

4. Avoid overheating, excessive sweating, and rechilling by loosening your clothing and not overdressing.

5. Drink ample fluids.

6. Protect the hands, feet, and head against frostbite and exposure.

7. Watch for early signs of frostbite and overexposure and treat immediately (see pages 153–154).

8. If it is too cold, exercise indoors or take a rain check that day.

Exercising in Polluted Air

There is an increasing concern about air pollution in our urban areas. There are three major pollutants that can affect your exercise.

1. *Carbon monoxide:* This gas displaces oxygen from the inhaled air and the red blood cells and reduces the amount of oxygen that can be transported in the body. This will impair athletic performance.

2. *Ozone:* Ozone is an oxidant that causes eye irritation, chest tightness, breathlessness, coughing, and nausea.

3. *Sulphur dioxide:* This is an upper-airway irritant that can cause discomfort in the throat and chest.

Many major cities have smog alert programs, and outdoor exercise should be avoided on these days. In general, you should avoid heavily traveled roads and rush-hour traffic when you exercise.

Exercising at High Altitudes

Exercising at high altitudes (above 7000 feet) places increased demands on the heart and lungs. Less oxygen is available as the altitude increases, making it difficult to deliver oxygen to the working muscles and thus decreasing the ability for peak performance, particularly in endurance events.

The body adapts quite rapidly, and partial acclimatization can be achieved in 3 to 5 days. Take time to acclimate to the new altitude. Heart and lung disease patients should use extreme caution when exercising at high altitude and should only do so if approved by a physician.

FIRST AID MEASURES

Frostbite

Signs and Symptoms

1. Early signs may include slightly flushed skin.

2. Color change to pale or ashen.

3. Pain may exist early and subside later. Often there is no pain.

4. Affected parts may feel intensely cold or numb.

First Aid

1. Protect affected parts from further exposure and injury.

2. Prevent chilling; add extra clothes or blankets.

3. Bring victim indoors.

4. Administer warm fluids but *no alcohol.*

5. Rewarm frozen area by immersion in warm water, not hot.

6. If water is not available, wrap gently in warm blankets.

7. *Do not rub the affected area.*

8. Elevate and try to gently exercise the affected part after it has been warmed.

Cold Exposure

Signs and Symptoms

1. Low body temperature

2. Shivering and numbness

3. Drowsiness and muscular weakness

4. Mental confusion and impaired judgment

5. Staggering and falling

6. Shock

7. Possibly heart fibrillation

First Aid

1. Administer artificial respiration if necessary.

2. Bring into warm room immediately.

3. Remove wet or frozen clothes.

4. Rewarm rapidly with warm blankets or a warm, not hot, tub of water.

5. If victim is conscious, give hot liquids but *no alcohol.*

6. Keep victim warm and treat for shock.

7. Transport to hospital.

Heat Exhaustion

Signs and Symptoms

1. Excessive sweating.

2. Temperature may be near normal.

3. Skin is pale or ashen and will feel cool and clammy.

4. Fainting may occur.

5. Victim may experience weakness, nausea, dizziness, or cramps.

First Aid

1. Victim should take sips of water (½ glass every 15 minutes). If victim vomits, discontinue.

2. Lie down; raise feet.

3. Loosen clothing.

4. Apply cool, wet cloths.

5. Fan victim or move to an air-conditioned room.

6. Transport to hospital.

Heat Stroke

Signs and Symptoms

1. Cooling system stops functioning.

2. Temperature is 105°F or higher.

3. Skin is hot, red, and dry.

4. *No sweating.*

5. Pulse is rapid and strong.

6. Victim may be unconscious.

7. Victim is in a life-threatening situation.

First Aid

1. Cool body quickly; prevent overchilling.

2. Undress victim, and sponge with cool towels or rubbing alcohol or apply cold packs or place in tub of cool water. Continue until temperature returns to normal.

3. When temperature has returned to normal, dry victim and fan or move to air-conditioned room.

4. Transport to hospital or call for emergency help.

Added Warnings

If you develop chest pain, an irregular heartbeat, or fluttering in your chest, stop exercising and seek medical attention. In addition, if any of the symptoms of heat stroke or heat exhaustion occur, get medical attention.

HOW DO YOU ENSURE THAT YOU DO THE EXERCISE?

We need to set short-term and long-term goals. The short-term goals are usually the need to accomplish the initial goal of 35 minutes of exercise and progress to the 45 to 60 minutes per session.

The long-term goals are achieving your ideal weight or body fat and fitness, as well as controlling or normalizing risk factors for blood pressure, heart disease, and diabetes.

To be successful with your exercise program, you need to satisfy two basic requirements: First, you need to know your target heart rate and then decide what form of aerobic exercise you want to do. Choose something you like to do or, for some of you, something you hate the least. It does not matter what you do, only that it is aerobic and that you do it for the prescribed period of time. Add variety if you need to. Second, and more important, you need to schedule your exercise. It should be planned in advance. Getting up in the morning with the best of intentions and saying to yourself that you are going to exercise that day does not guarantee anything. However, if you look at your schedule and plan to do it at a time of the day that you know is yours, then you will do it. Plan your exercise time the night before or, preferably, a week before. Keep a log on a weekly or monthly basis. It is always good motivation to look at what you have achieved.

SEVEN

Stress Awareness and Self-Management

Stress awareness and self-management have flourished in recent years. The causes of stress and the physical and emotional effect it has on us are becoming clearer.

Hans Selye called stress a specific bodily reaction to something out there which may be either stimulating and pleasant or noxious and harmful. It is any response to an event, demand, or stimulus which causes wear and tear on the mind and body.

Events good and bad may cause stress, the symptoms of which vary from one person to another. Upset stomach, fatigue, tight neck muscles, depression, and headaches are just a few of the common symptoms of stress. Stress may be linked to more serious and even fatal diseases, however, such as heart attacks, ulcers, and cancer.

Learning to manage stress is a three-part process:

1. Identify the symptoms and causes.

2. Learn skills to manage them.

3. Learn how to use those skills.

Stress may often be caused by events beyond your control, and then acceptance is the only way out. When it is caused by events within your control, the action taken will change the situation and probably relieve the stress.

WHAT IS STRESS?

Stress is different for everyone, and what is stressful for one may be harmless to another. It is a mismatch between the demands of our lives and the resources we have to deal with them. Stress is not the event but the reaction to the event.

The Physical Symptoms of Stress

Physical symptoms include the fight-or-flight reaction. When faced with sudden stress, e.g., seeing a snake in your pathway, adrenaline and other hormones are released into the bloodstream, and the following bodily reactions occur:

Pupils dilate.

The skin becomes pale.

Hands and feet become cooler as blood is diverted to the muscles to ready them for flight.

Muscle tension increases.

Digestion slows or stops.

Breathing rate increases.

Heart rate increases.

Perspiration increases to cool the body.

Sugar is released into the bloodstream from the liver.

Simply avoiding the snake and walking around it will remove the stress, and all these physiological responses will return to normal.

If we cannot make the stress go away, if we are stuck in a traffic jam with an important appointment only a few minutes away, the body is geared up with no place to go, and we cannot reverse the physical stress reaction. Thus we remain in a constant state of unproductive tension.

The fight-or-flight reflex is a primitive stress reflex that has had difficulty adapting to twentieth-century stresses. The resultant symptoms are called *distress*.

The Psychological Reactions to Stress

Events don't cause stress, but how you interpret them does. An individual's particular personality may predispose him or her to suffer certain stress-related diseases. Broadly speaking, the world can be divided into three groups of individuals: (1) type A personalities, (2) type B personalities, and (3) in-betweeners—those who flip-flop between the two.

Type A Personality: Harried Harry

The type A personality is characterized by individuals who live a self-imposed, stressful existence. They are engaged in a chronic struggle to achieve more in less and less time and are extremely competitive with a chronic sense of time urgency. The major characteristics of a type A are as follows:

1. *Time urgency:* Harried Harries don't like standing in lines, change lanes in traffic, always try to beat the traffic lights, interrupt you when you talk, and finish your sentences.

2. *Excessive achievement striving:* Time is the enemy and must be conquered, and it is an endless struggle. Deadlines are continuously set, and the type A is under constant time pressure. The deadlines are set to the exclusion of life's pleasures—self-punishment.

3. *Free-floating hostility:* In the constant struggle to achieve, the type A is very aggressive—every task is a challenge. The hostility is directed at everything that is in his or her path.

Type A behavior increases the risk of heart attacks only in the presence of the traditional risk factors, e.g., elevated cholesterol, high blood pressure, smoking, and diabetes. If none of these risk factors are present, there is no apparent increased risk for heart attack from being a type A.

Type B Personality: Laid-Back Linda

Type B people are laid back, relaxed, easygoing, and have a high self-esteem and confidence level. They appear to have no increased risk for heart attacks.

In-Betweeners

In-betweeners will exhibit traits of both personalities and don't usually have an increased cardiac risk. What you are will determine how you handle stress.

Is Stress Harmful?

Stress can hurt when it becomes a way of life and can lead to heart attacks, ulcers, cancers, and, possibly, other diseases. However, many people do their best work under stress, and it can be a powerful force for growth. We often learn or accomplish the most when we are forced to.

Thus we recognize the concept of positive and negative stress. Learning to recognize the symptoms and causes of stress will allow you to accept, cope with, or change the stresses. You need to learn how to balance and direct your energy. Instead of being a negative force, stress can become a powerful tool to help you achieve what you want.

WAYS OF COPING WITH STRESS

The first step in managing stress is to recognize it. Make a list of things that make you angry or upset and of things that make you happy, sad, frightened, unsure, startled, or excited. Any event that arouses strong emotions, positive or negative, has the potential to cause stress.

Next, consult Table 7-1 below to see which of the signs of stress it lists apply to you.

The first step in managing stress is to recognize it. Having thought about the causes and symptoms of stress, it is now important to log the stressor (the event causing the stress) and the stress response.

Set up a stress log as follows:

Stressor (what happened)   Stress response (how I reacted)

1. _____   1. _____

2. _____   2. _____

3. _____   3. _____

You must make two decisions regarding the stressor—how important it is and how you can control it.

Table 7-1   The Warning Signs of Stress

Physical	Emotional	Behavioral
Muscle tightness in neck and shoulders	Depression	Overeating
	Anger	Smoking and drinking
	Feelings of inevitability	Changes in sleeping habits
Pounding in heart		
Chest pain	Low self-esteem	Forgetfulness
Headaches	Apathy	Reckless driving
High blood pressure	Impatience	Drug use
Upset stomach		Negativity
Fatigue		
Cold, sweaty hands		
Eye strain		
Excessive sweating		
Constipation or diarrhea		
Nervous tics		
Rashes		
Tooth grinding		

Acceptance

Although it does no good to worry about things you cannot change, e.g., the weather, certain things will help you accept uncontrollable stress.

1. *Keep it in perspective:* We all worry about events that never come to pass. Always ask what else can be done, what is the worst possible outcome, and will you remember this 5 years from now?

2. *Use self-dialogue:* Talking to yourself often helps minimize the event. Someday you will look back at this and laugh, things could be worse, it's a learning experience, it has to get better, time is a great healer.

3. *Keep a positive attitude:* Try to smile when things are going wrong, even if it is rough. Focusing on the positive side will often lead to a more likely way out of the problem. Negative emotions will only make the situation worse.

Recognize if you are a type A, and try to modify some of the behavior traits. Try to accept that sometimes we fall short of our expectations; don't set unrealistic goals. Get involved in a regular, noncompetitive form of exercise, and consider problems as challenges. Always look for possibilities and creative solutions.

Counseling

If you feel completely alone, overwhelmed, or helpless, seek professional help. Seeking counseling is not a sign of weakness; it takes strength to realize you need help.

You may need to shop around for a counselor to find one that best suits your needs. Always ask what his or her approach to therapy is and how long it should take. Beware of therapists who try to hook you into unending therapy.

Exercise

There are many methods that can be used to cope with stress, and the simplest is physical exercise.

1. *Aerobic exercise:* Regular aerobic exercise is probably the easiest, simplest, and most effective method of stress relief available. When you are physically fit, your blood pressure, resting heart rate, and adrenaline levels are much lower. Your body is like a finely tuned machine, and if you are fit, getting good nutrition, and lots of sleep, you will have more energy and endurance to cope with stress.

   In addition, after 30 minutes of aerobic exercise, you begin to release endorphins in the brain which are naturally occurring, morphinelike, tranquilizing hormones. Endorphins will help to reduce stress and depression. They do not get rid of the underlying problem but may help you cope with it. Endurance sports, like running, swimming, and biking, induce a meditativelike state that is relaxing.

2. *Anaerobic exercise:* Exercises such as yoga and Tai Chi are also calming because they control breathing and induce a meditativelike state as well.

3. *Stretching:* Stretching relieves muscle tension and must be done gently so as not to be painful. Simple techniques that can be used to relax muscle tension while at your desk include shoulder rolls and raising the shoulders to your ears; side bends and reaching for the ceiling; circles with the feet and flexing your toes; and standing up and stretching to break the pattern of muscle tension.

Relaxation Techniques

Do you know how to relax? The traditional ways of relaxation with alcohol, cigarettes, watching TV, and eating may be more stress-inducing than relaxing.

True relaxation may reverse the physical effects of stress and will make you feel better, perform better, and think better. True relaxation is achieved very simply by some activity you enjoy that separates you from the stress, for example, reading a book, listening to music, playing a musical instrument, going to a movie, working in the garden, woodworking, knitting, or sewing. These simple events will take your mind off the stress if they are pleasurable for you.

Other ways of achieving a state of relaxation are included below. These techniques have to be learned. They are all effective, but each person needs to determine which technique best suits him or her.

1. *Simple muscular relaxation:* Progressive muscular relaxation training is perhaps the most widely used relaxation and stress control technique available today. It is easy to learn and quick.

   Assume a comfortable position either lying down or sitting in a chair, and with your eyes closed, systematically contract and relax each major muscle group in the body, working from head to toe. Becoming aware of the contrasting sensation of tension and relaxation in a muscle group is a crucial step in progressive muscular relaxation.

2. *Biofeedback:* With biofeedback the internal biological activity is measured, e.g., heart rate, blood pressure, and skin temperature. The object is to be able to control the biologic response, i.e., to achieve voluntary control over the activity. This requires repeated practice with the help of a biofeedback professional in order to recognize the symptoms and control them by measuring the response on a machine. This can be done with expensive, sophisticated machines or simply by using hand temperature as a guide. Place your hands on your cheeks, and if they are cooler than your cheeks you are stressed.

3. *Meditation:* Meditation is an Eastern art of relaxation that involves pure attention in the absence of cognitive processes. Simply put, it involves gaining mastery over one's attention. The incessant activity of the mind (going from one matter to the next) is stilled, and meditators achieve a sense of being that is completely distinct from their thoughts. It requires considerable practice and perseverance and needs to be taught to you by an experienced professional.

4. *Autogenic training:* The individual is taught via autogenic training to induce sensations that correlate the relaxation response by practicing a series of mental or physical exercises. A state of low arousal is achieved identical to the meditative state. It is achieved through passive concentration aided by visualization and imagery. Again, this needs to be taught by the appropriate professional.

In all four forms of stress control techniques, the individual seeks to develop harmony between the mind and body. The inability to relax is perhaps the most frequent complaint encountered by today's health-care provider. The ability to relax is innate—we are born with it. Yet there is evidence that modern men and women experience increasing estrangement from this marvelous capacity. Sustained distress and the concomitant failure to relax can become very costly.

Avoiding Stimulants

Stimulants such as caffeine, nicotine, cocaine, and amphetamines produce a ministress response by stimulating the fight-or-flight response and heightening the individual's stress level. Sugar may induce periods of elevated blood sugar followed by low blood sugar (hypoglycemia), raising and lowering your mood—the psychological roller coaster. Obviously, this induces lots of stress.

Managing Your Time

Probably our greatest failure is successful time management. Time is a resource that has to be managed:

1. Make lists of things to do that day, week, and month.

2. Prioritize your tasks, and do the most important ones when your energy is high.

3. Break down your tasks into manageable sizes.

4. Delegate where appropriate to those who are available to help, such as coworkers, spouse, kids.

5. Reduce paperwork by handling each piece of paper only once. Throw away junk mail without opening it.

6. Avoid time wasters. If someone drops in to chat, politely arrange to chat another time.

7. Admit when you have too many priorities, and ask for help.

8. Overcome procrastination. Set deadlines and meet them.

9. Learn to say no to new tasks. Don't feel guilty.

10. Manage the phone. Have calls screened, and ask when is the best time to return calls to avoid playing telephone tag. Always try to hang on rather than call back if the party is on the other line. Have the party you are holding for informed that you are waiting on the other line.

GETTING STARTED: THE S.M.A.R.T. PLAN

How do you turn all this into reality? A concrete, written plan will help keep you on course and increase your ability to get things accomplished. Start with realistic goals.

To begin, you need to get a picture of what you would like to happen in your life. It needs to be realistic and manageable. Prioritize those factors that cause stress and need work such as parenting, communication with children, or communication with coworkers. You need to be aware of the problems and develop appropriate action skills.

Failure of communication is at the root of many stress-related problems. Always try to be specific in the messages you send, and if you don't understand the messages you receive, clarify them rather than worrying about what they mean. Tell people exactly what you expect from them and what they can expect from you.

To help you set up a plan, you can use the S.M.A.R.T. plan:

Specific: Set a goal that addresses behavior and results, such as, "For the next month when I get stressed, I will use exercise or relaxation to cope."

Measurable: "My goal is to reduce the occasions when I feel stressed to fewer than one a day"—set milestones.

Agreed upon: Ask others to help you and support you; for example, let your boss know that you may need a few minutes to relax when under stress.

Rewarding: Behavior change should be firm. Reward yourself for achieving main goals and achieving milestones along the way. "For each week that I achieve my self-management goals, I will reward myself with an evening to myself doing exactly what I want."

Trackable: Keep track of your progress with a log, such as a stress log showing stressors and your response to them.

If you have the need, set up a contract with yourself, as follows:

I,_____ (your name), set the following *specific* and *measurable* goals for myself:_____

_____

The following people have *agreed* to help me in the following ways:

Person   Method of helping

_____   _____

_____   _____

_____   _____

I will give myself the following *rewards* at these milestones:

Reward   Milestone

_____   _____

_____   _____

_____   _____

I will keep *track* of my progress in the following way:

_____

_____

Signed _____

Witnesses _____

_____

Date _____

EIGHT

Countering Weight Gain with a Personalized Eating Plan

Some 34 million Americans are above their ideal weight, and 11 million are severely obese. In the Western world the average 35-year-old man gains 0.44 to 1.76 pounds of fat per year until the sixth decade.

People who have active lifestyles do not gain too much weight and maintain reasonably normal weights. There are multiple causes of obesity and many more short-term cures. Unfortunately, we have not found the long-term solution. We are constantly looking for the quick fix, and this creates more problems than it fixes.

The HealthMark program offers the most reasonable long-term solution to this problem.

THE HEALTH RISKS OF OBESITY

It was long thought that mild to moderate obesity brought no health risks with it. A National Institutes of Health panel recommended, however, that mild obesity be regarded as a disease because there are multiple biologic hazards at surprisingly low levels of excess fat, at only 5 to 10 pounds above desirable weight.

When fat is distributed centripetally (around the abdomen and chest), it is associated with more disease than fat around the arms and thighs, which is more genetic in origin.

The risks of obesity include the following:

1. Cardiovascular disease and atherosclerosis (heart attacks and strokes)

2. Strain on the heart muscle

3. High blood pressure

4. Diabetes (80 percent of adult-onset diabetics are obese)

5. Kidney disease

6. Gallstones

7. Impaired lung function

8. Increased risks for surgery and anesthesia

9. Degenerative joint disease (wear and tear)

10. Increased incidence of cancers of the uterus, breast, colon, and prostate

11. Psychological disturbances

Measuring Obesity

Defining obesity is best done by assessing percentage of body fat and the size and number of fat cells. The traditional height and weight tables are no longer valid because we find people who are overweight by these standards and yet have very low body fat percentages (bodybuilders, for example).

Percentage of Body Fat

Percentage of body fat is the most practical method of assessing obesity. It is best measured with underwater weighing methods, but this is impractical for most. The routine method with calipers used to pinch the fat is accurate enough unless you are severely obese. Other methods using electrical impedance and ultrasound are available, but their accuracy is in doubt.

Most health clubs are able to perform a body fat measurement for you, as can your local sports medicine center. Table 8-1 shows ideal body fat percentages for men and women of different body types.

We want to shoot for the average range. Massively obese people have 50 to 70 percent body fat.

Fat Cells

Fatness can also be measured by the number and size of the fat cells. Obese people may increase the size and number of fat cells. Nonobese people may have 25 to 30 billion fat cells, extremely obese people, 260 billion.

Weight reduction causes a decrease in the size of the fat cells but not the number, suggesting that obesity is difficult to cure. (It is difficult to measure fat cell size and number, and thus this discussion is more for an understanding of obesity rather than practical use.) Weight gain in adults increases the fat cell size but not the number. Fat cell size increases throughout infancy, childhood, and puberty. Fat cell numbers increase rapidly in the last trimester (three months) of pregnancy and the first year of life, then only gradually until the age of 10 and then again in adolescence.

You are stuck with the number of fat cells that develop, and fat babies often become fat adults. Excessive weight gain in pregnancy,

Table 8-1   Ideal Body Fat Percentages

Men	Women	Body Type
24+ %	29+ %	Obese
20–24%	27–29%	Very fat
17–20%	24–27%	Fat
13–17%	20–24%	Average
10–13%	17–20%	Trim
7–10%	14–17%	Skinny

bottle feeding, and early introduction to solid foods may be associated with obesity later in life.

Exercise early in life may aid in controlling the development of new fat cells and keeping down the cell size.

DIETS AND EXERCISE IN WEIGHT CONTROL

Consider this: If you ate an extra 100 calories per day without an increase in exercise to compensate for it, you would gain 10 pounds in a year and 100 pounds in 10 years—frightening isn't it?

Any effective weight-loss program must have a balance between calorie input and calorie output. Long-term results of all diet programs are only successful in 20 percent of the cases.

Weight loss or gain is a result of energy (calorie) input (I) and energy (calorie) output (O).

$$I = O \qquad \text{stable weight}$$
$$I > O \qquad \text{weight gain}$$
$$I < O \qquad \text{weight loss}$$

The best balance is less input and more output. For example, if you ate 100 less calories per day and burned 100 calories per day by exercise, the deficit is 200 calories, and this will result in a 21-pound weight loss in 1 year.

Diets and Weight Loss

Diets don't work. Eighty percent fail and lead to what has been called the "yo-yo syndrome."

It takes a 3500-calorie loss to lose 1 pound of fat. If you eat 1000 calories less per day, you should lose 7000 calories per week, or 2 pounds of fat. In fact, you lose more initially because after you deplete your carbohydrate stores (in muscle and liver), our best fuel, all the water held by the carbohydrate is lost. Each gram of carbohydrate holds 2.7 grams of water, and if the carbohydrate stores are filled, you can hold 2 to 4 pounds of water. This is why there is always such a rapid weight loss (water loss) on low calorie diets.

Most diets are very low in calories (under 1000) and are high in protein and low in carbohydrate. These diets will rapidly deplete carbohydrate stores, then break down your own muscle protein for energy, and only then fat. The metabolism of protein causes the production of uric acid, which leads to gout and kidney stones and also to the formation of urea. In an attempt to rid itself of these toxins, the body actually dehydrates itself by mobilizing fluids to excrete these toxins through the kidney. In addition, this causes a strain on the kidneys and may be associated with long-term kidney damage. Potassium loss with this may lead to heart rhythm disturbances. The metabolism of fat leads to the production of ketone bodies and a state called *ketosis* (an acidosis in the blood which can cause nausea, vomiting, fatigue, dizziness, and low blood pressure). Thus the weight loss that ensues is from water loss, muscle loss (protein), and some fat loss.

When you stop this very low calorie diet, the ketosis reverses rapidly, and, with resumption of carbohydrate intake, you will retain the water normally held in carbohydrate stores. In addition, the poor dehydrated body is like a sponge, sucking up fluid wherever it can. There is usually a rapid weight gain just from fluid retention. This leaves you psychologically defeated.

These diets (including liquid protein diets) don't work because they don't attempt to change the eating habits that made you obese. Thus when you have achieved weight loss, the old habits are usually renewed, and weight gain ensues.

Dieting also reduces the metabolic rate. As you reduce muscle mass on low calorie diets, the body's baseline energy needs (metabolic rate) are reduced—with severe calorie restriction, as much as 45 percent. The metabolic rate depends on the ratio of muscle to fat. Fat is metabolically inactive, and the more you have, the lower your metabolic rate. Thus as the diet progresses and the metabolic rate decreases, weight loss plateaus, and you become depressed and quit. Eating 600 to 800 calories per day and not losing weight is depressing.

When you regain weight, it comes back as fat (an increase in fat cell size), and the muscle lost is not readily replaced. Therefore, with each successive weight loss and gain (yo-yo), you gain more fat and lose more muscle. The overall effect of this higher fat/muscle ratio means it requires fewer calories to maintain the weight, and the new body requires less energy and a lower metabolic rate. Each time you go on a low-calorie diet it takes longer to lose the weight and you regain it faster and faster.

Exercise and Weight Loss

Exercise will increase the metabolic rate, increase lean body tissue (muscle), and increase the activity of enzymes that break down fat. We know that fat people may eat less, and they may be under-active. Children of obese adults are less active, and overweight children are less active.

The calorie deficits caused by exercise are cumulative, and when 3500 calories are burned, 1 pound of fat is lost. If you jog 30 minutes a day, you will burn 300 calories and will lose 1 pound in 12 days and 30 pounds in a year (see Table 8-2). Regularity of exercise is the key. The combination of mild dietary restriction and exercise is clearly the best.

Factors Affecting Weight Loss

When calorie intake is below the daily energy requirement, the initial decrease in body weight occurs primarily from water loss as the carbohydrate stores are depleted.

With a 1000-calorie restriction per day and moderate exercise, we find that the initial weight loss (1 to 3 days) is water (70 percent) and a little fat (25 percent). By days 11 to 13, fat loss is 69 percent, protein (muscle) 12 percent, and water 19 percent. By days 21 to 24, fat loss is 85 percent and protein 15 percent.

On ketogenic, or starvation, diets one-third of the weight loss is fat, two-thirds, muscle. On mixed diets (carbohydrate and protein), weight loss is two-thirds fat and one-third muscle. On mixed diets and exercise there is a net gain of muscle and a loss of fat. Diet and exercise obviously achieve the optimal results of reducing fat stores and building muscles.

Table 8-2   Calories Burned with Exercise per Hour

Type of Exercise	Body Weight (lbs)			
	125	170	205	230
Bicycling, 10 mph	218	296	357	401
Bicycling, 18 mph	312	463	559	625
Bicycling, racing	576	783	945	1059
Golf	289	398	475	532
Hiking, 40-lb pack, 3 mph	342	462	558	630
Racquetball	606	824	995	1116
Rowing machine	684	924	1116	1260
Running, 11.5-min mile	460	625	755	846
Running, 9-min mile	657	894	1079	1210
Running, 8-min mile	709	963	1163	1304
Running, 7-min mile	770	1056	1275	1434
Running, 6-min mile	859	1167	1409	1580
Skiing, cross-country, level	487	662	799	896
Skiing, cross-country, uphill	933	1269	1532	1718
Skiing, downhill	486	654	786	888
Snow shoeing, 2–5 mph	450	612	738	834
Soccer	450	606	732	804
Squash	722	981	1185	1329
Swimming, pleasure, 25 yd/min	300	408	492	552
Swimming, backstroke, 30 yd/min	264	360	432	492
Swimming, backstroke, 40 yd/min	420	564	684	768
Swimming, breaststroke, 30 yd/min	360	486	594	1080
Swimming, breaststroke, 40 yd/min	480	648	786	888

(continued)

Table 8-2   Calories Burned with Exercise per Hour
(*Continued*)

Type of Exercise	Body Weight (lbs)			
	125	170	205	230
Swimming, butterfly, 50 yd/min	588	792	954	1080
Swimming, crawl, 20 yd/min	240	324	390	438
Swimming, crawl, 50 yd/min	534	720	870	978
Tennis, recreation	192	252	318	360
Tennis, competitive	348	468	564	636
Walking, 2 mph	174	240	288	324
Walking, 4–5 mph	330	450	540	606
Waterskiing	390	528	636	720
Weight training	402	534	648	732
Circuit training, free weights	293	398	480	339
Circuit training, Hydrafitness	450	611	738	827
Circuit training, Nautilus	313	426	514	576
Circuit training, Universal	395	537	648	727

Source: Adapted from W. M. McArdl, F. I. Katch, V. L. Katch, *Exercise Physiology*, 2d ed., Lea and Febiger, Philadelphia, 1985; E. W. Bannister and S. R. Brown, "The Relative Requirements of Physical Activity," in H. B. Falls, ed., *Exercise Physiology*, Academy Press, New York, 1968; C. F. Consalszio, P. E. Johnson, and L. J. Pecora, *Physiological Measurements of Metabolic Functions in Man*, McGraw-Hill, New York, 1963, pp. 331–322; P. E. Allen, J. M. Harrison, B. Vance, *Fitness for Life: An Individualized Approach*, W. M. C. Brown, Dubuque, Iowa, 1978.

The net result of increasing the muscle-fat ratio should result in an increased metabolic rate.

How Many Calories Should We Restrict?

In general, calorie restriction should be mild and done by reducing the fat intake and eating more carbohydrates. Fat and alcohol intake (our most calorically dense foods at 9 calories per gram and 7 calories per gram, respectively) add unnecessary empty calories.

The best way to determine how much you need to eat is to determine your basal metabolic rate. This is defined as the number of calories burned per day to maintain your weight and carry out your regular bodily functions.

This is best estimated by the following formula: Your body weight times your level of activity equals your basal metabolic rate (BMR). To represent level of activity, use 10 to 12 for minimal or no physical activity (a sedentary desk job), 13 to 15 for moderate physical work, and 16 to 18 for heavy physical work (construction workers, farmers). For example, a 150-pound clerk will have a BMR of $150 \times 10 = 1500$ calories.

In addition, you need to add the number of calories burned with exercise on a daily basis (see Table 8-2) and add these to the total to estimate total daily calorie requirements.

The total number of calories needed on a daily basis is the number needed to maintain an ideal body weight. If you want to lose weight, reduce the calorie intake and exercise. For example, a 150-pound sedentary woman has a BMR of 1500. If she runs 3 miles per day, she burns an additional 300 calories, increasing her total calorie requirement to 1800 calories per day. To lose weight she must eat less or exercise more or preferably, both. In general, women should eat 1200 to 1500 calories per day when dieting and men between 1500 and 1800 calories, always combined with exercise. The secret to permanent weight loss is exercise (and mild calorie restriction).

Women do not lose weight as quickly as men. Women who have been on many low calorie diets (yo-yos) have an abnormally high fat-muscle ratio with a depressed metabolism. I have seen women who maintain weight on 600 to 800 calories of food per day and increase weight eating 800 to 900 calories. This can make life miserable and requires lots of patience and resolve to overcome. The only effective method is exercise to raise the metabolic rate and burn calories and slowly increase the calories eaten to a normal level. This often involves weight gain before weight loss occurs, but this is mostly muscle gain as fat loss progresses. A real weight loss may take a few weeks, but as long as fat loss (loss of inches) occurs, then you are progressing well. It takes lots of courage and perseverance and encouragement to push through this phase, and weight loss is generally slow at a pound per week or every other week. You have to go through this in order to restore your metabolism to its normal level of activity.

Work out your BMR taking all these factors into account, and then begin your mild calorie restriction and exercise program for a few weeks and judge the effect. Women should lose 1 to 2 pounds per week and men 2 to 4 pounds per week. This eventually slows down to 1 pound per week and then 1 pound every other week until the desired weight (estimated by your body fat) is achieved.

A general rule of thumb is 1 pound per week until the desired level is achieved. It is faster in the beginning and slower at the end.

People who have severe obesity and eating disorders should begin the program as described above. However, they should never ignore the psychological aspects of their problem. Permanent weight loss will never be achieved unless we tackle the reasons for overeating. They may include depression, escape from dealing with sexuality, and many other deep-seated psychological disorders. Psychotherapy may be an integral part of the approach to treatment along with the exercise and good eating habits.

A PERSONALIZED EATING PLAN

To lose weight (fat) and maintain this loss, you need to develop a plan you can live with that includes eating normally with a regular exercise program. The eating plan must allow you to eat enough to feel satisfied and prevent hunger and yet mildly restrict calorie intake. The exercise program must be tailored to your capabilities and needs (see Chapter 6), yet burn 1800 to 2000 calories per week for cardiovascular protection (that is, 400 calories per day exercising 5 days a week, or 350 calories per day exercising 6 days a week).

Three meals per day is the key. You need to spread your total calories over the course of the day so that you don't overeat at any one meal. Skipping breakfast and/or lunch will cause you to overeat at night, and this is when you burn the least calories because you are inactive. Most of the calories eaten at night are stored as fat.

Eat most of your calories during the day when you burn most of them, and try to spread the calorie intake evenly over the three meals. Never miss a meal.

There is an old saying: Breakfast like a king, lunch like a prince, and dine like a pauper, and you will never be fat.

Counting calories is discouraged—it is tedious and not very effective in permanent weight loss. However, you need to become familiar with the calorie content of most of the foods you eat so that you can keep yourself within the desired range.

Eliminating fat and alcohol removes a large portion of unnecessary calories, but even healthy, HealthMark choices can have excess calories; for example, a large whole wheat bagel can have up to 300 calories; nuts and avocados may have good oil but lots of calories as well.

The personalized eating plan (PEP) (see Appendix B) will help you design your own eating plan based on low fat, low cholesterol, high fiber foods. It will help you become aware of the calorie cost of different foods so that you can choose the appropriate portion sizes.

The first step is to determine your calorie requirements (as above), and this should not be an exact figure but rather a range. Then subtract your calories to produce weight loss from calorie restriction and those burned with exercise. A total calorie deficit of 500 calories per day for the average person is adequate. This should produce a loss of 1 pound per week (7 days × 500 calories = 3500 calories), and as mentioned before, it will occur faster in the beginning and slower in the end. The bookkeeping of weight loss is not an exact science.

The calorie deficit should come more from exercise than calorie restriction.

Remember, women tend to lose weight more slowly than men because they have a higher fat-muscle ratio than men.

In the tables in Appendix B you will find examples of calorie ranges of foods and portion sizes to help you work out your "routine" way of eating.

In Appendix B I have also laid out a 7-day eating plan using 1200-, 1500-, and 1800-calorie programs as examples.

You Can Still Eat and Lose Weight

There is no need to restrict your calories to any great extent. As mentioned, you should develop a lifestyle that you can live with. On this nutritional program you will be surprised at how much food you can eat and yet still lose weight. You will reduce consumption, or cut out some high calorie foods (fat and other empty calories such as sugar and alcohol), and eat much greater quantities of lower calorie foods such as grains, cereals, vegetables, breads, and pastas. All the foods that you thought were traditionally fattening are in fact good to eat, for example, pasta, potatoes, rice, and bread.

When you go to a restaurant and someone orders a steak and says, "Hold the baked potato; I'm on a diet," you will be able to tell them that they have it the wrong way around. A steak is 70 to 80 percent fat (of its calories) and has about 800 calories in a half-pound portion. A medium-sized baked potato with no fat added to it in the form of cream or butter is only 1 percent fat and has 70 calories. It does not make sense; you should eat two or three potatoes and send the steak back.

Two alcoholic drinks have about 300 calories, and the bowl of peanuts you eat adds another 800 calories, as each nut is 70 percent fat. This is 1100 calories you may consume as a predinner snack. It takes 9 to 10 miles of running to burn those calories off. If you cut the fat out of your diet, you will eliminate a large source of unnecessary calories and won't have a weight problem.

The calorie programs outlined are more for the people who need discipline in their eating rather than as a strict calorie guide. Use them as examples of how to put together a day's or a week's eating so you can develop regular habits.

Putting It All Together the HealthMark Way

You need to develop regular patterns of eating and exercise to be successful. Regular patterns will soon become habit, and when you have achieved this, you have won.

EXERCISE

Plan what you want to do and then schedule the time to do it. You will not exercise unless you make appointments with yourself. Be jealous of this time. It is going to make you feel good, so why give it to someone else? Plan to do your exercise at a time of the day that you know is going to be yours, not when other things usually crop up so that you can't do it. Push yourself to do the exercise so that if you miss a day after a few months of regular exercise and you wonder why you don't feel as good that day, you will realize that you missed the workout. Then you are hooked.

NUTRITION

Learn to eat three meals per day, and learn what to eat at each meal so that making the right choices becomes second nature.

Breakfast

A good bowl of high fiber cereal (hot or cold) with some fruit and skim milk takes care of a large portion of your fiber and calcium needs for the day. A cup of coffee with some wheat toast and jam compliments the meal. When you have the time, you can make the yolkless eggs, pancakes, or French toast. Breakfast is an important meal and does not take a long time to prepare. Learn which cereals are good and which you like, and from there on it is easy.

Lunch

In the United States, lunch is our smallest meal, whereas in Europe it is the main meal of the day. The European way is a healthier way of eating, because you ought to eat most of your calories at a time of the day when you are most active. Don't eat a heavy meal and then go to bed as you burn very few calories in your sleep, and thus most of these calories will be stored as fat.

It is not socially possible for most of us to eat our main meal at midday, and so we should eat a meal that is light. Save the 6 ounces of animal protein for dinner and eat soup and salad, or pasta, or fruit, yogurt, and bread (bagels or rolls). You can eat small amounts of animal protein in your salad or on your sandwich (1 to 2 ounces), just don't make the animal protein the main dish. Chinese food (stir-fry or steamed) is also a good light lunch, because there are lots of vegetables and small amounts of animal protein.

Dinner

Dinner is the main meal for most of us. Here you should eat the 6 ounces of animal protein (chicken, fish, or low fat beef or game) with salad, vegetables, and starch (rice or potatoes) and have fruit for dessert. Once a week you should not eat any animal protein for dinner and go vegetarian. You can eat pasta, lasagna, or stir-fry. This will make up for any excess cholesterol eaten during the rest of the week.

Snacks

Snacks should be eaten during the course of the day as needed. Fruit, crackers made with the good oils, bread sticks, bagels, and vegetables (carrot sticks) always make good snacks. If you can afford the calories, a peanut butter (natural-style peanut butter without bad fat added to it) and jelly sandwich is all right. Remember, 1 tablespoon of peanut butter has about 100 calories because it has a lot of fat even if it is good, monounsaturated fat.

Developing regular eating patterns will ensure that you are successful in your quest for a healthy lifestyle. Developing these patterns takes time, so be patient. Learn to eat the right foods most of the time, and the little indiscretions (10 percent time) won't amount to anything.

STRESS MANAGEMENT

Learn to recognize the stressors in your life as well as the stress responses you have. This is half the battle in learning to cope with stress. Learn techniques to relax (such as exercise), and if you still cannot control your stress, then seek professional help from a stress counselor.

Learn to make change slowly. Don't expect to achieve a complete lifestyle change in a few days. Set realistic goals and be patient. A complete lifestyle change takes months or years to perfect, and perfection is learning to blend the new habits into your life so that your risk factors are eliminated.

USING HEALTHMARKS AS A GUIDE

HealthMarks is a program designed to help you and your health professional monitor your progress. It is a points system that allows you to grade your HealthMark lifestyle to see how well you are doing.

In attempting to grade the effectiveness of your lifestyle change, you need to follow hard data such as changes in blood lipids, body weight, and blood pressure. In addition, if your cholesterol is not lowered within 6 months, or your lipid profile is still abnormal, or your blood pressure elevates again or does not go down, or your weight does not change, this system of HealthMarks will allow you to grade your lifestyle change prior to embarking on additional or alternative treatments such as medication.

In most cases, it will allow you to monitor your progress so that you can achieve a steady state. Some of you will want to monitor your progress continuously, and others may just want to monitor it 1 week per month. It is important to monitor yourself periodically to assess how well you are doing.

HealthMarks for Exercise

HealthMarks are given for exercise and nutrition and combined into daily and then weekly totals (see Table 9-1).

Table 9-1   HealthMarks for Exercise

	Your Score
Did you warm up and stretch?	+ 1
Did you exercise less than 20 minutes?	+ 0
Did you exercise 20 to 25 minutes?	+ 2
Did you exercise 26 to 30 minutes?	+ 3
Did you exercise 31 to 35 minutes?	+ 5
Did you exercise 36 to 40 minutes?	+ 6
Did you exercise 41 to 45 minutes?	+ 7
Did you exercise 46 minutes or more?	+ 7
Did you cool down and stretch after your workout?	+ 2

Note: Total points available on a daily basis = 10. Total points available on a weekly basis = 70.

The daily maximum in exercise HealthMarks is 10, and the weekly maximum is 70. However, you should only be exercising a maximum of 6 days a week for 60 HealthMarks. If you are exercising more, you are doing it for some reason other than cardiovascular protection, perhaps training for endurance events or stress management.

The optimum HealthMarks needed for cardiovascular protection is enough exercise to burn 1800 to 2000 calories per week, which roughly translates into 18 to 20 miles of fast walking or jogging per week. This requires a minimum frequency of four to five times a week of exercise of at least 35 to 45 minutes per session. The range for average exercise is about 28 to 35 HealthMarks per week.

20–27	Should be better
28–35	Average
36–45	Excellent
46–60	Outstanding
61+	Too much exercise

HealthMarks for Nutrition

The best score for nutrition points is the highest possible, and your maximum nutritional score on a weekly basis is 70. (See Table 9-2.) There is a weekly bonus of 1 mark if you are at your ideal weight or are losing weight steadily. The maximum for a week is 71 HealthMarks.

Total HealthMarks for Overall Lifestyle

Table 9-3 is the combined weekly total of exercise and nutritional HealthMarks, and your score here is the most important indication of your overall compliance.

Table 9-2   HealthMarks for Nutrition

	HealthMark	Goal
Do you eat 3 meals a day?	+ 2	Regular meals
Do your HealthMark meals include the following?		
6 oz (or less) lean protein (low fat beef, skinless chicken, fish, etc.) or egg whites	+ 1	
16 oz skim milk (2 glasses) or low fat or nonfat yogurt or calcium supplements	+ 1	Calcium
4 or more servings of whole wheat bread, whole grains, oatmeal, oat bran, barley, dried beans	+ 1	Fiber
At least 2 servings of citrus fruit, melon, berries, baked potato, tomato	+ 1	Fiber and vitamin C
At least 2 servings of broccoli, cauliflower, cabbage, brussels sprouts, dark-green leafy vegetables, dark-orange vegetable, and fruit	+ 1	Fiber, vitamin C, carotene
1 tsp or less of salt per day (including sodium in foods)	+ 1	Salt reduction
2 cups (or less) regular coffee per day or water-processed, decaffeinated coffee	+ 1	Caffeine reduction
Fewer than 2 drinks of alcohol per day (1.5 oz hard liquor or 10 oz wine or 2 bottles of beer)	+ 1	Alcohol reduction
Subtract 1 point for any of the following:		
More than 6 oz of animal protein per day	− 1	

Table 9-2   HealthMarks for Nutrition (*Continued*)

	HealthMark	Goal
High fat meats: Hot dogs, bacon, sausage, lunch meats	− 1	
Cheese, butter, sour cream, ice cream, other high fat dairy products	− 1	
Egg yolks	− 1	
Fried foods	− 1	
Fast foods	− 1	
Salty, fatty snacks (e.g., chips, crackers)	− 1	
Baked goods made with egg yolks and saturated fat (e.g., cake, pie, pastry, cookies, croissants, muffins, granola)	− 1	
Chocolate, candy made with fat (e.g., caramels)	− 1	
More than 2 tbsp of salad dressing (oil-based) or more than 1 tsp of soft or liquid margarine	− 1	
Weekly bonus point:		
Are you at target weight and body fat percentage or are you losing ½ to 1½ lbs per week?	+ 1	

Note: Maximum daily HealthMarks for nutrition = 10.

Bad news for smokers: Continued smoking requires that you subtract 5 HealthMarks per day.

We don't reward you for doing too much. Above 130 you will have excellent dietary compliance, but you will be exercising too much. Watch out for the effects of chronic fatigue and over-training.

Table 9-3   Total HealthMarks

HealthMarks	Comment
60–90	Bare minimum—needs improvement
91–110	Average
111–120	Excellent
121–131	Outstanding
132–141	Too much exercise

APPENDIX A

Stretching Exercises

Stretching should always be done as part of the warm-up and cool down. Warm-up stretches should be light and easy because when muscles are cold they are susceptible to tearing. Never stretch to the point of pain, and stretch the muscles you will use most in the exercise you plan to do.

Cool down stretching should be longer. Once your muscles are warmed up from exercise, they can be stretched easier and longer without fear of injury. This stretching program should involve all muscle groups.

A consistent stretching program will prevent injury and muscle soreness and will increase flexibility of muscles and joints. Never bounce when you stretch. Always hold the stretch for 10 to 20 seconds and breath easily while you stretch.

Once you have developed a consistent stretching program, you can do it less frequently to maintain the flexibility of your muscles and joints. However, stretching is always a very relaxing part of the exercise and for this reason should not be omitted to save time.

STANDING STRETCHES

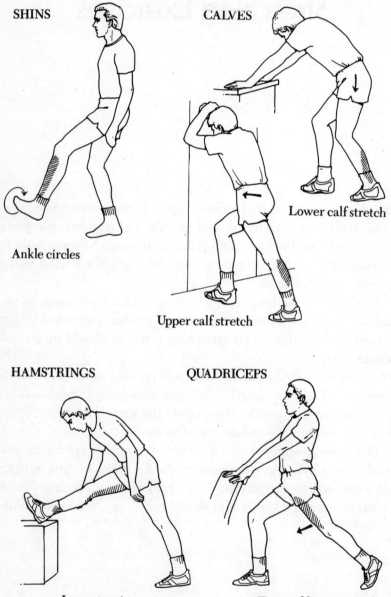

SHINS

Ankle circles

CALVES

Lower calf stretch

Upper calf stretch

HAMSTRINGS

Leg extensions

QUADRICEPS

Forward lunges

TORSO

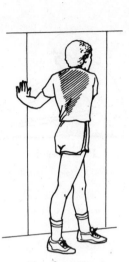

Trunk twisters

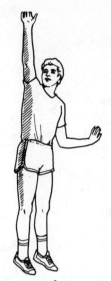

Torso reaches

SHOULDERS AND ARMS

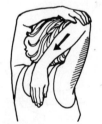

Shoulder stretch A
(behind the head)

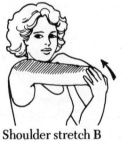

Shoulder stretch B
(across the front)

NECK

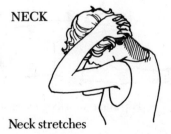

Neck stretches

FLOOR STRETCHES

HAMSTRINGS

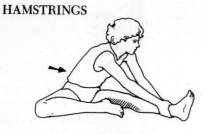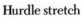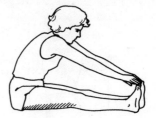

Hurdle stretch   Pike stretch

BACK

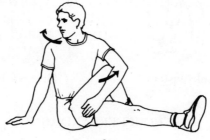

Spinal twist

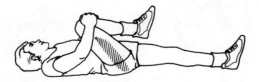

Lower back stretch

QUADRICEPS

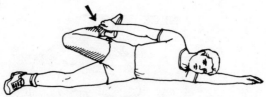

Hip and quadricep extensor

A P P E N D I X   B

The HealthMark Eating Plan and Sample Menus

The HealthMark eating plan is a 7-day dietary plan designed for those people who need structure. Use the plan to get started; once you are familiar with the types of foods eaten, substitutes can be made easily to create variety.

You will become aware of the overall calorie cost of various foods. However, you should not count calories. Eating the correct portion sizes and keeping to low fat foods will naturally reduce the calorie intake without any major bookkeeping effort. (See pages 178–179 to calculate which plan is best for you.)

Women should be at 1200 to 1500 calories per day and men at 1500 to 1800 calories per day. You should have plenty to eat and not go hungry; you should not feel as though you are on a diet—only that you have changed your way of eating.

The menu plans are based on recipes found in the recipe section (Appendix C). Please refer to the recipes as you work your way through the menu plan.

	How Much		
What to Eat	*1200-Cal. Diet*	*1500-Cal. Diet*	*1800-Cal. Diet*
Lean meat, fish, or skinless poultry	4 oz	6 oz	6 oz
Complex carbohydrate	5 servings	7 servings	8 servings
Vegetables	4 servings	5 servings	6 servings
Fruits	4 servings	4 servings	6 servings
Milk	2 servings	2 servings	2 servings
Fats	3 tsp	4 tsp	5 tsp

Monday

1200 Calories	Calories	1500 Calories	Calories	1800 Calories	Calories
BREAKFAST		**BREAKFAST**		**BREAKFAST**	
1 cup shredded wheat	140	1 cup shredded wheat	140	1 cup shredded wheat	140
½ banana	50	½ banana	50	1 banana	100
1 cup skim milk	90	1 cup skim milk	90	1 cup skim milk	90
	280	1 slice whole wheat toast	70	1 slice whole wheat toast	70
		1 tsp jam	16	1 tsp jam	16
			366		416
LUNCH		**LUNCH**		**LUNCH**	
2 cups salad	50	3 cups salad	75	3 cups salad	75
¼ cup kidney beans	55	⅓ cup kidney beans	80	⅓ cup kidney beans	80
1 tbsp Vinaigrette Dressing[1]	100	1⅓ tbsp Vinaigrette Dressing[1]	135	2 tbsp Vinaigrette Dressing[1]	200
1 slice whole wheat bread	70	1 slice whole wheat bread	70	1 baked potato	220
1 large apple	100	1 cup vegetable soup	50	¼ cup cottage cheese	45
	375	1 large apple	100		620
			510		
DINNER		**DINNER**		**DINNER**	
4 oz Red Snapper[2]	135	6 oz Red Snapper[2]	200	6 oz Red Snapper[2]	200
1 cup steamed broccoli	50	1 cup steamed broccoli	50	1 cup steamed broccoli	50
½ cup brown rice	100	1 cup brown rice	200	1 cup brown rice	200
1 slice French bread	70	1 slice French bread	70	1 slice French bread	70
½ cup strawberries	25	1 cup strawberries	50	1 cup strawberries	50
½ cup nonfat vanilla yogurt	90	½ cup nonfat vanilla yogurt	90	½ cup nonfat vanilla yogurt	180
	470		660		750
Total	1125	Total	1536	Total	1786

[1]See recipe for Vinaigrette Dressing, page 209.
[2]See recipe for Snapper in Tomato-Wine Sauce, page 233.

Tuesday

1200 Calories

	Calories
BREAKFAST	
1 cup oatmeal	140
2 tbsp raisins	50
1 cup skim milk	90
	280
LUNCH	
Grilled chicken sandwich:	
4 oz grilled chicken breast	200
2 oz whole wheat bun	140
Sliced tomatoes and lettuce	25
Dijon mustard	—
1 nectarine	50
	415
DINNER	
2 cups salad	50
1 tbsp Vinaigrette Dressing[1]	100
1 cup eggless pasta	180
¼ cup Marinara Sauce[2]	25
½ cup grapes	50
1 cup skim milk	90
Total	495
	1190

1500 Calories

	Calories
BREAKFAST	
1 cup oatmeal	140
2 tbsp raisins	50
1 cup skim milk	90
½ cup orange juice	60
	340
LUNCH	
Grilled chicken sandwich:	
4 oz grilled chicken breast	200
2 oz whole wheat bun	140
Sliced tomatoes and lettuce	25
Dijon mustard	—
1 cup skim milk	90
1 nectarine	50
	505
DINNER	
2 cups salad	50
1 tbsp Vinaigrette Dressing[1]	100
2 cups eggless pasta	360
¾ cup Marinara Sauce[2]	75
1 cup diced fresh fruit	100
Total	685
	1530

1800 Calories

	Calories
BREAKFAST	
1 cup oatmeal	140
2 tbsp raisins	50
1 cup skim milk	90
½ cup orange juice	60
2 slices whole wheat toast	140
2 tsp jam	32
	512
LUNCH	
Grilled chicken sandwich:	
4 oz grilled chicken breast	200
2 oz whole wheat bun	140
Sliced tomatoes and lettuce	25
Dijon mustard	—
1 cup vegetable soup	50
1 cup skim milk	90
1 nectarine	50
	555
DINNER	
2 cups salad	50
1 tbsp Vinaigrette Dressing[1]	100
2 cups eggless pasta	360
¾ cup Marinara Sauce[2]	75
1 slice French bread	70
1 cup diced fresh fruit	100
Total	755
	1822

[1]See recipe for Vinaigrette Dressing, page 209.
[2]See recipe for Marinara Sauce, page 220.

Wednesday

1200 Calories	Calories
BREAKFAST	
1 eggless bagel (whole wheat)	160
1 tbsp peanut butter	100
1 tsp jam	16
1 orange	50
1 cup skim milk	90
	416
LUNCH	
1½ cups assorted fruit plate	150
½ cup 1% cottage cheese	90
3 rye crisps	75
	315
DINNER	
4 oz Bombay Lime Chicken[1]	200
1 cup steamed broccoli	50
½ cup rice	100
½ cup nonfat frozen yogurt	100
	450
Total	1181

1500 Calories	Calories
BREAKFAST	
1½ eggless bagels (whole wheat)	240
1 tbsp peanut butter	100
2 tsp jam	32
1 orange	50
1 cup skim milk	90
	512
LUNCH	
2 cups assorted fruit plate	200
½ cup 1% cottage cheese	90
3 rye crisps	75
	365
DINNER	
6 oz Bombay Lime Chicken[1]	300
1 cup steamed broccoli	50
½ cup rice	100
1 whole wheat roll	80
½ cup nonfat frozen yogurt	100
	630
Total	1507

1800 Calories	Calories
BREAKFAST	
1½ eggless bagels (whole wheat)	240
1 tbsp peanut butter	100
2 tsp jam	32
1 orange	50
1 cup skim milk	90
	512
LUNCH	
2 cups assorted fruit plate	200
½ cup 1% cottage cheese	90
3 rye crisps	75
1 cup orange juice	120
	485
DINNER	
6 oz Bombay Lime Chicken[1]	300
1 cup steamed broccoli	50
½ cup rice	100
1 whole wheat roll	80
1 cup nonfat frozen yogurt	200
	730
Total	1727

[1]See recipe for Bombay Lime Chicken, page 225.

Thursday

	1200 Calories	Calories	1500 Calories	Calories	1800 Calories	Calories
BREAKFAST						
	1⅓ cups bran flakes	140	1⅓ cups bran flakes	140	1⅓ cups bran flakes	140
	1 cup berries	50	1 cup berries	50	1 cup berries	50
	1 cup skim milk	90	1 cup skim milk	90	1 cup skim milk	90
			1 slice whole wheat toast	70	1 English muffin, whole wheat	140
			1 tsp jam	16	1 tsp jam	16
		280		366		436
LUNCH						
	1 medium baked potato	220	1 medium baked potato	220	1 medium baked potato	220
	¼ cup Salsa (for the potato)[1]	10	¼ cup Salsa (for the potato)[1]	10	¼ cup Salsa (for the potato)[1]	10
	¼ cup 1% cottage cheese	45	¼ cup 1% cottage cheese	45	½ cup 1% cottage cheese	90
	1 cup salad	25	2 cups salad	50	3 cups salad	75
	½ tbsp Vinaigrette Dressing[2]	50	1 tbsp Vinaigrette Dressing[2]	100	1⅓ tbsp Vinaigrette Dressing[2]	135
					1 large apple	100
		350		425		630
DINNER						
	4 oz Halibut Provencal[3]	140	6 oz Halibut Provencal[3]	210	6 oz Halibut Provencal[3]	210
	½ cup steamed carrots	25	½ cup steamed carrots	25	½ cup steamed carrots	25
	½ cup steamed peas	50	½ cup steamed peas	50	½ cup steamed peas	50
	½ cup brown rice	100	1 cup brown rice	200	1 cup brown rice	200
	1 cup skim milk	90	1 cup grapes	100	1 cup grapes	100
	½ cup grapes	50	1 slice Angel Food Cake[4]	100	1 slice Angel Food Cake[4]	100
	1 slice Angel Food Cake[4]	100				
		555		685		685
Total		1185		1476		1751

[1]See recipe for Salsa, page 207.
[2]See recipe for Vinaigrette Dressing, page 209.
[3]See recipe for Halibut Provencal, page 230.
[4]See recipe for Angel Food Cake, page 245.

Friday

1200 Calories

	Calories
BREAKFAST	
1 cup oat bran	140
½ sliced banana	50
1 cup skim milk	90
	280
LUNCH	
Turkey sandwich:	
2 slices whole wheat bread	140
2 oz sliced turkey	100
Lettuce and tomato	25
Dijon mustard	—
½ cup grapes	50
	315
DINNER	
1 slice (2½" × 4½" × 2" deep) Lasagna[3]	290
2 cups salad	50
1 tbsp Vinaigrette Dressing[4]	100
½ cup Instant Sorbet[5]	110
1 cup skim milk	90
	640
Total	1235

1500 Calories

	Calories
BREAKFAST	
1 cup oat bran	140
½ sliced banana	50
1 HealthMark muffin[1]	105
2 tsp jam	32
1 cup skim milk	90
	417
LUNCH	
Turkey sandwich:	
2 slices whole wheat bread	140
2 oz sliced turkey	100
Lettuce and tomato	25
Dijon mustard	—
1 cup grapes	100
1 cup skim milk	90
	440
DINNER	
1½ slices Lasagna[3]	435
2 cups salad	50
1 tbsp Vinaigrette Dressing[4]	100
½ cup Instant Sorbet[5]	110
	710
Total	1577

1800 Calories

	Calories
BREAKFAST	
1 cup oat bran	140
½ sliced banana	50
1 HealthMark muffin[1]	105
2 tsp jam	32
1 cup skim milk	90
½ cup orange juice	60
	477
LUNCH	
1 cup Gazpacho[2]	50
Turkey sandwich:	
2 slices whole wheat bread	140
2 oz sliced turkey	100
Lettuce and tomato	25
Dijon mustard	—
1 cup grapes	100
1 cup skim milk	90
1 frozen fruit bar	70
	575
DINNER	
1½ slices Lasagna[3]	435
3 cups salad	75
1⅓ tbsp Vinaigrette Dressing[4]	135
½ cup Instant Sorbet[5]	110
	755
Total	1807

[1]See recipes for HealthMark muffins, pages 237–238.
[2]See recipe for Gazpacho, page 216.
[3]See recipe for Lasagna, page 219.
[4]See recipe for Vinaigrette Dressing, page 209.
[5]See recipe for Instant Sorbet, page 246.

Saturday

1200 Calories	Calories	1500 Calories	Calories	1800 Calories	Calories
BREAKFAST		BREAKFAST		BREAKFAST	
2 5-in HealthMark pancakes[1]	140	3 5-in HealthMark pancakes[1]	210	3 5-in HealthMark pancakes[1]	210
1 tbsp maple syrup	50	1 tbsp maple syrup	50	1 tbsp maple syrup	50
½ cup orange juice	60	½ cup orange juice	60	1 cup orange juice	120
1 cup skim milk	90	1 cup skim milk	90	1 cup skim milk	90
	340		410		470
LUNCH		LUNCH		LUNCH	
Cold pasta salad:		Cold pasta salad:		Cold pasta salad:	
¾ cup cold cooked pasta	135	1 cup cold cooked pasta	180	1 cup cold cooked pasta	180
1 cup mixed steamed vegetables	50	1 cup mixed steamed vegetables	50	1 cup mixed steamed vegetables	50
1 tbsp Vinaigrette Dressing[2]	100	1 tbsp Vinaigrette Dressing[2]	100	1 tbsp Vinaigrette Dressing[2]	100
1 tbsp Parmesan cheese	25	1 tbsp Parmesan cheese	25	1 tbsp Parmesan cheese	25
½ cup grapes	50	½ cup grapes	50	1 cup grapes	100
				1 slice whole wheat bread	70
	360		405		525
DINNER		DINNER		DINNER	
4 oz Oven-Poached Fish[3]	200	6 oz Oven-Poached Fish[3]	300	6 oz Oven-Poached Fish[3]	300
½ cup brown rice	100	½ cup brown rice	100	½ cup brown rice	100
½ cup steamed asparagus	50	½ cup steamed asparagus	50	½ cup steamed asparagus	50
1 cup salad	25	2 cups salad	50	2 cups salad	50
½ tbsp Vinaigrette Dressing[2]	50	1 tbsp Vinaigrette Dressing[2]	100	1 tbsp Vinaigrette Dressing[2]	100
½ cup nonfat frozen yogurt	100	½ cup nonfat frozen yogurt	100	1 cup nonfat frozen yogurt	200
	525		700		800
Total	1225	Total	1515	Total	1795

[1]See recipes for HealthMark pancakes, pages 248–249.
[2]See recipe for Vinaigrette Dressing, page 209.
[3]See recipe for Oven-Poached Fish, page 229.

Sunday

1200 Calories	Calories	1500 Calories	Calories	1800 Calories	Calories
BREAKFAST		**BREAKFAST**		**BREAKFAST**	
½ whole wheat English muffin	70	1 whole wheat English muffin	140	1 whole wheat English muffin	140
1 tsp jam	16	1 tsp jam	16	1 tsp jam	16
omelette:		omelette:		omelette:	
3 egg whites[1]	60	3 egg whites[1]	60	3 egg whites[1]	60
½ cup chopped onions and tomatoes	25	½ cup chopped onions and tomatoes	25	½ cup chopped onions and tomatoes	25
½ oz part-skim milk mozzarella cheese	35	1 oz part-skim milk mozzarella cheese	70	1 oz part-skim milk mozzarella cheese	70
		½ grapefruit	50	1 grapefruit	100
1 cup skim milk	90	1 cup skim milk	90	1 cup skim milk	90
	296		451		501
LUNCH		**LUNCH**		**LUNCH**	
1 cup Gazpacho[2]	50	1 cup Gazpacho[2]	50	1 cup Gazpacho[2]	50
1 cup nonfat fruit yogurt	200	1 cup nonfat fruit yogurt	200	1 cup nonfat fruit yogurt	200
½ eggless whole wheat bagel	80	1 eggless whole wheat bagel	160	1 eggless whole wheat bagel	160
1 peach	50	1 peach	50	2 peaches	100
	380		460		510
DINNER		**DINNER**		**DINNER**	
1½ cups Chicken with Peanuts[3]	250	1½ cups Chicken with Peanuts[3]	250	2 cups oz Chicken with Peanuts[3]	320
1 cup brown rice	200	1 cup brown rice	200	1 cup brown rice	200
½ cup Instant Sorbet[4]	110	½ cup Instant Sorbet[4]	110	1 cup Instant Sorbet[4]	220
	560		610		740
Total	1236	Total	1521	Total	1751

[1]Use HealthMark Egg Substitute; see recipe on page 247.
[2]See recipe for Gazpacho, page 216.
[3]See recipe for Spicy Chicken with Peanuts, page 227.
[4]See recipe for Instant Sorbet, page 246.

A P P E N D I X C

Favorite HealthMark Recipes

This recipe section is taken from the HealthMark cookbook, *Cooking for a Healthier Everafter* written by Susan Stevens, MS, RD, the nutrition director at HealthMark.

These recipes have been developed for your enjoyment as well as your health and are a testimonial to the fact that healthy food can look good and taste great. They are low in fat, cholesterol, and sodium and high in fiber. They conform to the HealthMark guidelines.

Once you become familiar with the HealthMark style of cooking, you can modify some of your existing recipes. It is amazing how many old favorites can be modified and still look and taste the same.

Enjoy your new cooking style and the good health it brings.

TIPS ON RECIPE MODIFICATION

Reducing Fat and Cholesterol

1. Buy lean cuts of meat and trim all visible fat. Use grass-fed beef or "good" or "select" grade.

2. Avoid organ meats, which are very high in cholesterol.

3. Broil, bake, roast, poach, or stir-fry meat, poultry, and fish instead of pan-frying or deep-fat frying.

4. Sauté in nonstick cookware using a minimum of oil (1 to 2 teaspoons) or sauté with broth, wine, or water. (Chefs call this "sweating.")

5. Serve poultry, fish, whole grains, dried beans, peas, and lentils more often.

6. Cook poultry without the skin; reduce cooking time by one third to one half to prevent overcooking.

7. Make stock, soups, and stews ahead of time; chill, and remove all hardened fat. If there is no time to do this, skim off as much fat as possible, then add several ice cubes. Fat will congeal and cling to the ice cubes, which can then be discarded.

8. Reduce the amount of fat in baked goods by one-third to one-half. Use vegetable oil (safflower oil is the least saturated) or soft margarine whenever possible. Quick breads, muffins, pancakes, and waffles turn out perfectly well made with oil rather than a more saturated fat such as butter, shortening, or stick margarine. Soft margarine can be substituted for butter or stick margarine in many recipes.

9. Use nonfat or 1 percent dairy products (milk, yogurt, or cottage cheese). Use evaporated nonfat milk in soups, sauces, and baking.

10. Substitute nonfat yogurt or puréed cottage cheese for sour cream.

11. Substitute 3 tablespoons unsweetened cocoa powder and 1 tablespoon oil for 1 ounce baking chocolate.

12. Reduce nuts in a recipe; use only ¼-⅓ cup.

13. In baking, substitute 1 to 2 egg whites for each whole egg.

Reducing Salt

1. Eliminate or reduce salt in all recipes except yeast breads where salt is necessary to control growth of the yeast.

2. Use onion and garlic powders instead of salts.

3. Use salt-free canned vegetables and soups.

4. Use light (reduced sodium) soy sauce—sparingly.

5. Use salt-free beef and chicken broth. For a more concentrated flavor, boil to reduce by half. Be sure to defat canned broth by chilling until fat hardens, then skimming.

6. Rinse canned tuna, salmon, shrimp, crab, or clams to reduce salt content.

Reducing Sugar

1. Reduce sugar by one-third to one-half. In cookies and cakes, replace the eliminated sugar with nonfat dry milk.

2. When sugar is reduced, enhance flavor with spices (cinnamon, nutmeg, or cloves) and extracts (vanilla, almond, orange, or lemon.)

3. Substitute brown sugar or honey for white sugar; use less because the flavor is sweeter.

4. When reducing sugar in quick breads, cakes, and cookies, use fruits which add sweetness naturally such as raisins, dried apricots, dates, or bananas.

Adding Fiber

1. Use whole wheat flour whenever possible. As it is heavier than white flour, use less: ⅞ cup whole wheat flour to 1 cup white flour.

2. Add wheat bran or oat bran to baked goods, cereals, casseroles, soups, and pancakes.

3. Use potatoes unpeeled ("country style") whenever possible in soups, stews, or oven-fries.

4. Use more vegetables, whole grains (bulgur, corn, barley, and oatmeal), dried beans, split peas, and lentils.

A P P E T I Z E R S

ROB'S CREAM CHEESE

1 cup nonfat cottage cheese

Puree cottage cheese in blender or food processor until smooth. Spoon into coffee filter or cheesecloth. Place in a strainer, then suspend over a bowl. Cover and place in refrigerator for 24 to 48 hours.

Excess moisture will drain/evaporate, and a creamy spread will remain. Use on bagels, toast, quick breads, or as a base for dips.

YIELD: 1 CUP

HEALTHMARK SOUR CREAM

1 cup nonfat cottage cheese
¼ cup nonfat yogurt, buttermilk, or nonfat milk
1 tbsp lemon juice

Puree all ingredients in blender or food processor until *very* smooth.

Use as a topping for baked potatoes. May also be substituted for mayonnaise in tuna or chicken salad.

YIELD: ABOUT 1¼ CUPS

HOMEMADE ("FAT-LESS") TORTILLA CHIPS

1 pkg corn tortillas **or**
  1 pkg whole wheat flour tortillas
water
garlic, onion, or chili powder (optional)

Brush tortillas one at a time with water. If desired, sprinkle lightly with garlic, onion, or chili powder. Cut into six to eight wedges.

Arrange tortilla wedges on a nonstick or lightly oiled baking sheet. Bake at 425° for 5 to 7 minutes, turn and bake another 5 to 7 minutes or until crisp. Repeat until all chips are baked.

PITA CHIPS

whole wheat pita bread, split in half
safflower or olive oil
part-skim Parmesan cheese
poppy or sesame seeds

Brush pita bread *lightly* with oil. Sprinkle *lightly* with Parmesan, then with poppy or sesame seeds. Cut into eight wedges. Arrange on a baking sheet. Bake at 350° until crisp, about 5 to 10 minutes.

Pita chips may also be prepared without oil. Cut into wedges, then bake until crisp.

TEX-MEX DIP

3 ripe avocados, peeled
2 tbsp lemon juice
¼ tsp pepper
1 cup plain nonfat yogurt
½ cup light mayonnaise
1 1⅛-oz package taco seasoning mix
2 10½-oz cans jalapeño-flavored bean dip (no lard)
1 bunch green onions with tops, chopped
2 3½-oz cans pitted ripe olives, drained and coarsely chopped
4 oz lowfat cheddar cheese, shredded
*   tortilla chips*

In a medium bowl mash avocados with lemon juice and pepper. In a small bowl combine yogurt, light mayonnaise, and taco seasoning mix.

To assemble: Spread bean dip on a large, shallow serving platter;

top with avocado mixture, then spread with yogurt mixture. Sprinkle with chopped onions, tomatoes, olives, and shredded cheese.

Serve chilled or at room temperature with tortilla chips.

YIELD: 16 APPETIZER SERVINGS

BLACK BEAN DIP

1 *onion, chopped*
1 *tbsp olive oil*
1 *clove garlic, minced*
1 *15-oz can black beans, drained*
1 *tsp celery seed, crushed*
1–2 *tbsp Worcestershire sauce*
¼ *tsp hot pepper sauce (optional)*
chopped fresh cilantro

Sauté onion and garlic in olive oil until softened, but not brown, about 5 minutes. Cool slightly. Combine with beans and remaining ingredients in a food processor or blender. Process until smooth.

Pour into a saucepan and simmer over low heat for 15 to 25 minutes or until of dipping consistency.

Serve hot or cold garnished with chopped cilantro. Serve with homemade tortilla chips or fresh vegetables.

YIELD: 1½ CUPS

FRESH SALMON TARTARE

2 *lb fresh salmon fillet, cut into chunks*
¼ *cup minced fresh parsley*
2 *tbsp capers, rinsed and drained*
2 *tbsp chopped fresh chives*
2 *tbsp olive oil*
3 *tbsp fresh lemon juice*
2 *tsp Dijon mustard*
dash hot pepper sauce

Coarsely chop salmon in food processor or by hand; do not puree. Transfer to a medium bowl and blend in parsley, capers, and chives. In a separate bowl, whisk together oil, lemon juice, mustard, and hot pepper sauce. Add to salmon and toss lightly; do not mash. Chill for 2 hours.

Serve with pumpernickel or black rye bread.

YIELD: 3 CUPS

SALSA

2 or 3 green onions
1 clove garlic
1 28-oz can salt-free whole tomatoes **or**
    5 to 6 fresh tomatoes, cored and chopped
¼ cup chopped green chiles (or jalapeños)
¼ cup fresh cilantro leaves
1 tsp oregano
¼ tsp cumin

In a blender or food processor chop onions and garlic. Add remaining ingredients and process until coarsely chopped.

Use as a topping for baked potatoes, a dip for fresh vegetables, or as a topping for grilled chicken or fish. Also serve with freshly made Tortilla Chips (page 204) or spooned over an egg white omelette.

YIELD: ABOUT 2 CUPS

CAPONATA

1 large eggplant, diced
1 onion, sliced
¼ cup olive oil
6 tomatoes, cored and diced
2 stalks celery including tops, diced
½ cup sliced black olives, rinsed and drained
2 tbsp capers, rinsed and drained
2 tbsp **each** sugar and red wine vinegar
½ tsp pepper

Sauté eggplant and onion in olive oil until lightly browned. Add tomatoes and celery. Cover and cook over low heat for 15 minutes. Add olives, capers, sugar, vinegar, and pepper. Cover and simmer an additional 15 minutes.

Chill before serving.

SERVES: 4 TO 6

HUMMUS

  ¼ *cup sesame seeds or 2 tbsp tahini*
  1 *15-oz can garbanzo beans, rinsed and drained*
  3 *tbsp lemon juice*
  1 *tbsp olive oil*
  1–2 *cloves garlic, crushed*
  ¼–½ *tsp cumin (optional)*

In a dry skillet toast sesame seeds, stirring frequently, until golden. Combine all ingredients in a food processor or blender and pulse on and off until well chopped. Then process for 30 to 45 seconds until light and fluffy. If mixture is too thick add water, one tablespoon at a time, until desired consistency is reached.

Serve with whole wheat pita bread wedges, lowfat crackers, breadsticks, or raw vegetables.

YIELD: 2 CUPS

SALADS

CREAMY CUCUMBER DRESSING

  1 *unpeeled cucumber, seeded*
  1½ *cup nonfat cottage cheese*
  ¼ *cup plain nonfat yogurt*
  ¼ *cup chopped onion* **or** *2 green onions, thinly sliced*
  1 *tsp dill*

Combine all ingredients in blender or food processor. Puree until very smooth. Use as a salad dressing or as a sauce for salmon.

YIELD: 1¾ CUPS

MUSTARD SAUCE

  1½ cup plain nonfat yogurt
    2 tbsp Dijon mustard
1–2 tbsp red wine vinegar
    1 tsp soy sauce
    1 clove garlic, minced
  ½ tsp marjoram **or** tarragon

Combine all ingredients and blend well. Cover and chill. Use as a topping for baked potatoes, as a salad dressing, or as a dip for fresh vegetables.

YIELD: 1½ CUPS

VINAIGRETTE DRESSING

  ¼ cup **each** red wine vinegar and water
  ¾ cup olive oil
  ¼ tsp **each** salt and pepper
  ½ tsp **each** paprika and dry mustard
  1 clove garlic, minced
  1 tsp parsley
  ½ tsp **each** basil and oregano

Whisk all ingredients together. Store in a tightly covered jar. Shake well before serving.

YIELD: 1½ CUPS

ZERO CALORIE DRESSING

½ cup salt-free tomato juice
2 tbsp lemon juice **or** red wine vinegar
1 tbsp onion, minced
1 tsp dried parsley
1 clove garlic, minced

mustard, horseradish, basil, oregano: optional

Combine all ingredients in a jar with a tightly fitting lid. Shake well before serving.

YIELD: ABOUT ¾ CUP

CHICKEN PASTA SALAD PRIMAVERA

1 cup safflower oil
⅔ cup red wine vinegar
1 tsp sugar **or** apple juice concentrate
1 clove garlic, minced
½ tsp **each** salt and pepper
1 tsp Dijon mustard
1 tsp Worcestershire sauce
1 tsp paprika

½ lb eggless pasta (e.g., bow ties), cooked and drained
2 cups skinless, cubed, cooked chicken
¼ lb fresh mushrooms, sliced
2 cups broccoli, cooked and chopped
1 10-oz package frozen peas, thawed
½ pint cherry tomatoes, sliced in half
1 cup chopped celery
¼ cup chopped green onions
1 8-oz can water chestnuts, sliced (optional)
2 tbsp dried basil
½ tsp pepper

Mix together first eight ingredients for the dressing. Pour ⅓ cup of dressing over cooked pasta while it is still warm. Chill for at least 3 hours or overnight.

Add the chicken, vegetables, basil, and ⅓ cup of dressing to the pasta and toss. Serve on lettuce-lined plates. Serve remaining dressing on the side.

SERVES: 5 TO 8

variation:
Substitute seafood (such as scallops, crab, and/or salmon) for chicken.

RAINBOW COLE SLAW

1 *small head of green cabbage, finely shredded*
1 *small head of red cabbage, finely shredded*
2 *unpeeled Golden Delicious apples, cored and diced*
4 *carrots, shredded*
2 *green* **or** *red peppers, diced*
1 *red onion, thinly sliced*

⅔ *cup frozen orange juice concentrate, thawed*
⅓ *cup raspberry* **or** *red wine vinegar*
2 *tsp dry mustard*
½ *tsp ginger*
1 *clove garlic, minced*

In a large bowl combine cabbages, apples, carrots, peppers, and onion.

In a small bowl whisk together ingredients for dressing. Combine with cabbage mixture and toss to mix thoroughly. Cover and chill before serving.

SERVES: 10 TO 12

MARINATED CUCUMBERS

¾ *cup white vinegar*
¼ *cup sugar* **or** *apple juice concentrate*
2 *unpeeled cucumbers*
3 *green onions, thinly sliced*
½ *tsp dill*

Score cucumbers with a fork; remove seeds and slice thinly. Mix vinegar and sugar in a saucepan. Bring to a boil to allow sugar to dissolve. Mix with cucumber, green onion, and dill. Marinate several hours or overnight.

SERVES: 4 TO 6

INDONESIAN RICE SALAD
(from Alfalfa's Market)

¼ *lb snow peas*
2 *cups cooked rice (brown* **or** *white)*
2–3 *green onions, thinly sliced*
1 *cup chopped celery*
½ *cup chopped fresh parsley*
1 *cup chopped green pepper*
1 *8-oz can water chestnuts, sliced*
¼ *lb bean sprouts, washed and drained*
1 *cup diced pineapple*
1 *unpeeled apple, seeded and chopped*
1 *cup halved red* **or** *green grapes*
½ *cup unsalted cashews*
½ *cup raisins*
¼ *cup toasted sesame seeds*

½ *cup orange juice concentrate, thawed*
¼ *cup safflower oil*
1 *tsp* **each** *ginger and grated orange peel*

2 *tsp tamari*
1 *clove garlic, minced*

Steam snow peas for 2 to 3 minutes. Rinse under cold water, then drain well. In a large bowl combine with remaining ingredients and mix well.

To prepare dressing: Blend together orange juice concentrate, oil, spices, tamari, and garlic. Pour over salad and toss gently, blending well.

SERVES: 10 TO 12

FRENCH POTATO SALAD

2 *lb unpeeled new potatoes*
4 *tbsp low-sodium, defatted chicken broth*
4 *tbsp wine vinegar*
1 *tsp dry mustard*
  freshly ground pepper to taste
2–3 *tbsp olive oil*
½ *cup thinly sliced green onions* **or** *chopped red onions*
¼ *cup chopped fresh parsley*

Steam potatoes for 20 to 30 minutes or until just tender. Cool, then slice. Place in a large mixing bowl. Add chicken broth and mix gently.

Blend together vinegar, mustard, and pepper. Pour over warm potatoes and blend well. Let potatoes rest for 10 minutes, then stir in olive oil, onions, and parsley.

Serve at room temperature.

SERVES: 6 TO 8

MARINATED VEGETABLE SALAD

Assorted fresh vegetables to total 4–5 cups; chop or slice into bite-sized pieces:

> *broccoli, steamed just until tender*
> *cauliflower, steamed just until tender*
> *carrots*
> *green beans*
> *celery*
> *mushrooms*
> *zucchini*
> *jicima*
> *cherry tomatoes, halved*
> *red, white, or green onion*
> *⅓–½ cup vinaigrette dressing (page 209)*

In a large bowl combine vegetables with dressing; toss to coat evenly. Cover and refrigerate overnight. Serve chilled.

Serves: 4 to 6

variation:
Add 2 cups cooked eggless pasta and/or 1 cup cooked, dried beans (e.g., kidney or garbanzo).

PINK AND GREEN PASTA SALAD

> *8 oz eggless pasta (e.g., rotini)*
> *½ lb cooked baby shrimp*
> *1 10-oz package frozen peas, thawed and drained*
> *4 green onions, thinly sliced*
> *1 cup sliced celery, tops included*
> *½ cup dry roasted, unsalted cashews*
>
> *1 cup plain nonfat yogurt*
> *1–2 tbsp light mayonnaise*

1 tbsp lemon juice
1 tsp dill weed

Cook pasta according to package directions. Drain and cool to room temperature. Mix with shrimp, peas, vegetables, and nuts.

Blend together last four ingredients and toss with pasta mixture. Chill before serving.

SERVES: 4

TABOULI

1 cup bulgur, uncooked
2 cups hot water
3 tomatoes, cored and chopped
1 cucumber, seeded and chopped
6 green onions, thinly sliced
½ cup chopped fresh parsley
2 tbsp fresh mint, minced, **or** 2 tsp dried mint
¼ cup lemon juice
2 tbsp olive oil
½ tsp oregano
¼ tsp celery salt
½ tsp pepper

Combine bulgur and water in a bowl and soak 1 hour. Drain well.

Add remaining ingredients to bulgur, mixing well. Chill for 2 hours before serving. Serve cold or at room temperature. May be served in a scooped-out tomato or in pita bread.

additions:

¼ cup sunflower seeds (dry roasted, unsalted)
1 cup garbanzo or kidney beans
1 6½-oz can water-packed tuna
plain nonfat yogurt
½ cup grated carrots and/or jicima

S O U P S

FISHERMAN'S STEW

  1 *tbsp olive oil*
  3 *cloves garlic, minced*
  2 *onions, chopped*
  2 *carrots, chopped*
  2 *stalks celery, chopped*
  ¼ *tsp crushed fennel seeds* **or** ⅛ *tsp crushed saffron threads*
  1 *16-oz can salt-free Italian tomatoes, chopped*
  ½ *cup dry white wine*
  ½ *tsp crushed red pepper*
  ½ *tsp thyme*
  1 *bay leaf*
  1 *8-oz bottle clam juice*
  1 *cup water*
  1 *lb fish fillets (sole, flounder, orange roughy, or halibut), cut into bite-sized pieces*
  1 *tbsp anise-flavored aperitif (such as Pernod or Ricard)*

Sauté garlic and onions in oil until soft. Add carrots, celery, fennel, tomatoes and juices, wine, pepper, thyme, bay leaf, clam juice, and water. Bring to a boil, then simmer, covered, about 15 minutes or until vegetables are just tender. Add fish; cook about 4 to 5 minutes. Stir in aperitif. Serve immediately.

SERVES: 4

GAZPACHO

  2 *unpeeled cucumbers, seeded*
  5 *tomatoes, cored*
  1 *onion, white* **or** *red*
  1 *green pepper, seeded*

1 *clove garlic*
¼ *cup* **each** *red wine vinegar and olive oil*
¼ *tsp* **each** *celery salt and cumin*

Coarsely chop vegetables. Puree in blender or food processor.
Blend in vinegar, oil, celery salt, and cumin.
Chill before serving.

SERVES: 6 TO 8

HEARTY LENTIL SOUP

1½ *cups lentils*
1 *tbsp olive oil*
1 *onion, chopped*
1 *clove garlic, minced*
2 *cups salt-free, defatted chicken* **or** *beef broth*
4 *cups water*
1 *cup* **each** *sliced carrots and celery*
1 *cup chopped cabbage*
1 *unpeeled potato, diced*
1 *tsp Liquid Smoke*
½ *tsp* **each** *thyme and marjoram*
   ground pepper to taste

Wash and drain lentils. In a 4-quart pan, sauté onion and garlic
in olive oil until soft. Add lentils and remaining ingredients. Bring
to a boil. Skim if necessary. Reduce heat and simmer, covered, for
45 to 60 minutes until lentils and vegetables are tender. Stir occasionally. Remove bay leaf before serving.

YIELD: ABOUT 2 QUARTS

MINESTRONE

  1 cup Great Northern beans, uncooked
  1 tbsp olive oil
  1 large onion, chopped
  1 leek, washed well and sliced
2–3 cloves garlic, minced
  ¼ cup chopped fresh parsley
  1 tsp **each** basil, oregano, and thyme
  1 cup sliced celery, including tops
  1 green **or** red pepper, chopped
  1 cup sliced carrots
  1 cup green beans, cut into 1-in pieces
  1 28-oz can salt-free Italian tomatoes, chopped
  1 cup zucchini, sliced
  1 tsp salt
  1 cup uncooked small pasta, eggless (e.g., small macaroni
    shells)
  1 10-oz package frozen peas, thawed

Soak beans according to directions on page 221. Discard soaking water and add 6 cups fresh water. Sauté onion, leek, and garlic in olive oil. Add to beans along with parsley, basil, oregano, and thyme. Bring to a boil, then simmer, covered, 1 to 2 hours or until beans are tender, stirring occasionally.

Add remaining vegetables, salt, and pasta. Continue to simmer until tender, about 30 minutes.

Put ¼ cup peas in each soup bowl, then add hot soup. Sprinkle with 1 tablespoon part-skim Parmesan cheese if desired.

SERVES: 6 TO 8

PASTA

LASAGNA

½ *pound ground turkey or lean ground beef*
1 *onion, chopped*
2 *stalks celery (including tops), chopped*
2 *cloves garlic, minced*
1 *one-pound, 12-oz can crushed pear tomatoes*
1 *14-oz can pear tomatoes, chopped*
1 *12-oz can tomato paste*
2 *tsp basil*
1 *tsp oregano*
½ *tsp fennel seeds, crushed*
½ *tsp Lite Salt*
¼ *tsp thyme*
½ *tsp pepper*
    8 oz lasagna noodles (eggless), cooked without salt

cheese filling:
2 *cups low-fat ricotta (Gardenia)*
2 *cups 1 percent cottage cheese*
¼ *lb part-skim mozzarella, grated*
2 *tbsp chopped fresh parsley*
2 *egg whites*
⅓ *cup part-skim Parmesan cheese*

Cook ground turkey, onion, celery, carrots, and garlic in a skillet over medium heat until meat is no longer pink. Add tomatoes, tomato paste, herbs, salt, and pepper and simmer 30 minutes or until thickened.

Meanwhile, make cheese filling: In a large bowl combine ricotta, cottage cheese, mozzarella, egg whites, and parsley. Mix well and set aside.

Cook noodles al dente according to package directions, omitting salt. Set aside.

To assemble: Coat a 9-inch × 13-inch baking dish with cooking spray. Spread half the sauce on the bottom. Cover with half the noodles, then spread with the cheese filling. Cover with remaining noodles and sauce. Cover lightly with foil. Bake at 350° for 25 minutes. Uncover, sprinkle with Parmesan cheese and bake another 10 to 15 minutes.

SERVES: 10 TO 12

MARINARA SAUCE

1 onion, chopped
2 cloves garlic, minced
1 tbsp olive oil
½ lb mushrooms, sliced
1-2 carrots, grated
1-2 zucchini, grated
1 green or red pepper, chopped
2 28-oz cans salt-free tomatoes, chopped
¼ cup dry red wine (optional)
1 tsp **each** basil and oregano
¼ tsp thyme
¼ cup chopped fresh parsley

Sauté onion and garlic in olive oil until soft. Add mushrooms, carrots, zucchini, and green pepper; cook 3 to 4 minutes, stirring.

Add remaining ingredients and simmer, covered, for 45 to 60 minutes; stir occasionally. Serve over eggless pasta or use in lasagna.

YIELD: ABOUT 6 CUPS

BEANS

The delectable bean—a great source of complex carbohydrate, fiber, protein, iron, and vitamins. All this nutrition for about 100 calories per ½ cup; 1 ounce of steak—which is just a bite or two—contains the same number of calories with saturated fat and cholesterol as well.

Unfortunately the humble bean is often neglected because of the long cooking time required. But with some planning beans can assume a place of honor on your dinner table.

Proper soaking not only reduces cooking time but eliminates much of the gas many people suffer when eating beans. Cooking beans in fresh water is the key.

Cleaning: After discarding small stones and discolored or shriveled beans, rinse dry beans or peas in cold water.

Soaking (Quick method): In a large pan cover each cup of beans with 3 cups water. Bring to a boil and boil for 2 minutes. Cover and let soak for 1 hour. Discard water, and add fresh, 3 to 4 cups per cup of beans. Proceed with recipe. (Overnight soaking: In a large pan combine beans and water in the same proportion as above. Soak overnight. Discard water and replace with fresh water. Proceed with recipe.)

BEANS AND RICE

  1 *onion, chopped*
  2 *cloves garlic, minced*
  1 *green* **or** *red pepper, chopped*
  1 *cup carrots, chopped or grated*
  2 *zucchini, chopped or grated*
  1 *16-oz can salt-free kidney beans, undrained*
  ¼ *cup chopped fresh parsley*
  1 *tsp* **each** *basil and oregano*
    pepper to taste
  ½ *tsp salt*
  2 *tomatoes, cored and diced*
  5 *cups cooked brown rice*

Sauté onion, garlic, peppers, celery, carrots, and zucchini in oil until soft. Add beans, parsley, and seasonings. Cover and simmer 30 minutes. Stir in diced tomatoes. Serve over hot brown rice. Sprinkle with ⅓ cup part-skim Parmesan cheese if desired.

SERVES: 6

QUICK CHILE CON CARNE

½ cup chopped onion
½ cup chopped green pepper
½ lb lean ground beef **or** ground turkey
1 15-oz can salt-free tomato sauce
1 15-oz can salt-free whole **or** stewed tomatoes
2 15-oz cans salt-free kidney beans, drained
½–1 tsp chili powder
¼ tsp **each** cumin and pepper
¼ tsp dry mustard

Combine onion, green pepper, and crumbled ground beef or turkey in a plastic colander placed in a 2-quart glass casserole. Microwave on full power for 6 minutes, stirring every 2 minutes. Pour off drippings. Transfer mixture to casserole dish. Add remaining ingredients. Microwave on full power, covered, for 10 to 12 minutes, stirring halfway through cooking. Let stand, covered, for 5 minutes.

SERVES: 4 TO 6

FELAFEL

A great filling for a pita sandwich; use smaller size pita bread for appetizers.

4 cups cooked garbanzo beans (salt-free, if canned)
3 cloves garlic
1–2 stalks celery, including tops, chopped
½ cup chopped onion
2 egg whites
1–2 tbsp tahini (sesame seed paste) **or**
    1 tbsp olive oil
3 tbsp dry bread crumbs
½ tsp **each** cumin and turmeric
¼ tsp **each** cayenne and salt

Process beans in blender or food processor until smooth. Add remaining ingredients and process again until well mixed. Chill.

Form mixture into 1-inch balls (oil your hands if necessary to prevent batter from sticking). Place on lightly oiled or nonstick baking sheet. Bake at 350° until golden brown, about 15 minutes.

Serve hot in pita bread with sliced cucumber, sliced tomato, and alfalfa sprouts. Top with plain nonfat yogurt.

YIELD: ABOUT A DOZEN 1-INCH BALLS

VEGETABLE CHILI
Delicious served over brown rice

½ cup bulgur
1 cup hot water
1 red onion, chopped
1 white onion, chopped
1 tbsp olive oil
3 garlic cloves, minced
½ cup **each** chopped celery and carrot
1–2 tbsp chili powder
1–2 tbsp (or less, if desired) cumin
½ tsp cayenne pepper
2 tsp **each** basil and oregano
1 **each** yellow squash and zucchini, cubed
1 **each** green and red pepper, cubed
1 cup mushrooms, sliced
2 15-oz cans salt-free kidney beans, undrained
1 15-oz can salt-free tomatoes
¾ cup white wine **or** salt-free, defatted beef broth

Combine bulgur and hot water. Let soak 30 minutes to soften.

Sauté onions in oil until tender. Add garlic, celery, and carrots; sauté 3 to 4 minutes. Add chili powder, cumin, cayenne, basil, and oregano. Cook, covered, over low heat until carrots are almost tender.

Add yellow squash, zucchini, green and red peppers, mushrooms, bulgur, beans, tomatoes, and wine. Simmer, covered, 30 minutes or until vegetables are tender.

SERVES: 8

CHICKEN

BARBECUED OVEN-FRIED CHICKEN

2–3 *lb chicken parts, skinned*
  1 *cup Rice Krispies*
  1 *tsp chili powder*
 ½ *tsp garlic powder*
 ¼ *tsp dry mustard*
 ¼ *tsp celery seed, crushed*
 ¼ *tsp paprika*
 ½ *cup barbecue sauce (see page 225)*

Rinse chicken; pat dry with paper towels. Mix together Rice Krispies and seasonings. Brush each chicken piece with barbecue sauce and roll in cereal mixture to coat.

Arrange chicken in a lightly oiled 13-inch × 9-inch baking pan. Bake, uncovered, at 375° for 50 minutes or until chicken is tender and coating is crisp Do not turn.

SERVES: 6

BARBECUE SAUCE

  2 cups salt-free tomato sauce
½ cup molasses
½ cup cider **or** white vinegar
½ cup brown sugar **or** apple juice concentrate
¼ cup safflower oil
¼ cup chopped onion
  1 tbsp dry mustard
  1 tbsp Worcestershire sauce
  2 tsp paprika
½ tsp **each** pepper and garlic powder

In a medium saucepan, bring all ingredients to a boil. Simmer, uncovered, for 30 minutes stirring occasionally. Cool slightly, then pour into a jar, cover, and store in refrigerator.

YIELD: ABOUT 2 CUPS

BOMBAY LIME CHICKEN
(from The Canterbury Inn)

½ cup lime juice
  4 green onions, thinly sliced
¼ cup mint, chopped
¼ cup fresh cilantro, chopped
  1 tsp minced shallots
  1 clove garlic, minced
  1 tsp pepper
¾ cup olive oil
  4 chicken breasts, skinned

Combine all ingredients, except chicken breasts, and mix well. Pour marinade over chicken breasts and marinate for 1 hour.
Broil, brushing with marinade.

SERVES: 4

ORANGE-TERIYAKI CHICKEN

1 6-oz can frozen orange juice concentrate, thawed
¼ cup reduced-sodium soy sauce
2 tbsp chopped onion
½ tsp ground ginger (**or** 1 tsp fresh ginger)
½ tsp hot pepper sauce
6 chicken breasts, skinned

Combine all ingredients but chicken. Add chicken, coating each piece with marinade. Cover and marinate 3 hours or more in refrigerator.

Remove from marinade and broil until chicken is tender and cooked through.

SERVES: 6

ROAST CHICKEN

1 roasting chicken, skinned and excess fat removed
3 tbsp vinegar
3 tbsp olive oil
1 tbs juice
½ tsp **each** savory, sage, and basil
1 clove garlic, minced
12 oz fresh mushrooms

In a small saucepan, mix all ingredients except chicken and mushrooms. Bring sauce to a boil, stirring. Remove from heat. Dip mushrooms in sauce and set aside.

Brush chicken evenly with remaining sauce.

Place chicken on a rack in roasting pan. Roast at 375°, basting every 20 minutes, for 1 to 1½ hours or until chicken is done. Add mushrooms to pan during last 20 minutes.

SERVES: 4

SAGE VINAIGRETTE

(from the Augusta in the Westin Hotel)

2 tbsp sherry vinegar
1½ tbsp Dijon mustard
1 tbsp chopped fresh sage **or** 1 tsp dried sage
1 cup olive oil

Process vinegar, mustard, and sage in a blender or food processor. Slowly drizzle in oil with motor running until all is incorporated. Heat gently in a double boiler to 145° before serving.

Especially good on chicken. Use sparingly as this sauce is quite high in fat.

YIELD: ABOUT 1¼ CUPS

SPICY CHICKEN WITH PEANUTS

2 chicken breasts, skinned and boned
2 tsp safflower oil
1½-in slice fresh ginger, minced
1 clove garlic, minced
¼–½ tsp dried chili pepper (optional)
¼ cup dry roasted, unsalted peanuts
1 green pepper, sliced
1 onion, sliced
4 green onions, sliced into 1-in pieces
3 stalks celery, sliced on the diagonal
1 cup sliced mushrooms
2 cups precooked* chopped broccoli
1 cup precooked* sliced carrots
1 pkg frozen pea pods, thawed
1 tbsp reduced-sodium soy sauce
1 tsp dark sesame oil (optional)

Cut chicken into bite-sized pieces. Heat wok or skillet. Add 1 teaspoon oil; swirl to coat entire surface. Add ginger, garlic, and chili pepper. Stir-fry 1 minute. (Avoid breathing chili fumes.) Add chicken and peanuts; stir-fry 2 to 3 minutes or until chicken is done. Remove and drain on paper towels.

Add remaining teaspoon of oil. Stir-fry remaining vegetables (except pea pods) until tender crisp Add small amounts of water as needed to prevent sticking.

Add chicken, pea pods, and soy sauce. Stir-fry 1 minute. Drizzle in sesame oil. Serve over steamed brown rice.

SERVES: 6 TO 8

*To precook: Place chopped vegetables in plastic bag. Seal and cook in microwave 1 minute or steam for 3 to 4 minutes.

Other vegetables to add to the stir-fry are:
   zucchini
   red or green cabbage
   bok choy
   water chestnuts
   bamboo shoots
   bean sprouts (add along with chicken at last minute)

variations:
   After vegetables are stir-fried, add 1 to 2 cups cooked brown rice. Stir-fry until rice is heated than add chicken, pea pods, and seasonings.

   Substitute lean beef, scallops, orange roughy, monkfish, halibut, salmon, or other firm white fish for chicken.

   Substitute cubed tofu for chicken.

TANDOORI-STYLE CHICKEN

   5 garlic cloves
   1 1-in cube peeled ginger
   1 medium onion, cut into 8 wedges
   1 cup plain nonfat yogurt
   3 tbsp lemon juice
   1 tbsp olive oil
   2 tsp ground coriander
   1 tsp cumin

1 tsp turmeric
½ tsp pepper
¼ tsp cardamom
¼ tsp nutmeg
¼ tsp ground cloves
¼ tsp cinnamon
¼ tsp cayenne pepper
8 chicken pieces, skinned

chopped green onion
lemon wedges

Mince garlic in processor. Add ginger and mince. Add onion and mince. Add next twelve ingredients and puree. Transfer to bowl. Cut deep slashes in chicken pieces. Add to marinade, turning to coat well. Cover and refrigerate overnight.

Preheat broiler. Arrange chicken on broiler pan and broil about 3 inches from heat source, 5 minutes per side. Reduce oven temperature to 325°. Transfer chicken to lightly oiled baking dish. Bake until juices run clear when pierced with tip of sharp knife, basting frequently with marinade, 20 to 25 minutes. Garnish with green onion and lemon wedges.

SERVES: 4

FISH AND SEAFOOD

OVEN-POACHED FISH

¼ cup chopped onion
½ cup **each** sliced mushrooms and chopped celery
1 lb fish fillets
1 bay leaf
3–4 peppercorns
2–3 sprigs fresh parsley
¼ cup **each** white wine and water

Spread onion, mushrooms, and celery over bottom of a lightly oiled 8-inch × 8-inch baking dish. Place fish on top. Add seasonings, wine, and water. Bake at 350° for 20 minutes or until fish flakes easily with a fork. Drain and serve immediately.

SERVES: 4

HALIBUT PROVENCAL

   2 *halibut steaks, 6 oz each*
   1 *tbsp olive oil (or less)*
   1 *tomato, cored and diced*
   ½ *cup sliced fresh mushrooms*
   ¼ *cup* **each** *chopped onion and green pepper*
   ⅓ *cup dry white wine*
   1 *tbsp chopped fresh parsley*
   1 *clove garlic, minced*
   ⅛ *tsp salt*
   ¼ *tsp pepper*
   ⅛ *tsp thyme*
   1 *bay leaf*

Sauté halibut in oil until lightly browned. Add remaining ingredients. Bring to a boil, then simmer, covered, 10 to 15 minutes.

Remove fish and vegetables; keep warm. Cook liquid until reduced to about ¼ cup. Pour over fish and vegetables and serve.

SERVES: 2

SALMON (SWORDFISH) ORIENTAL

   ½ *cup orange juice*
   1 *tbsp reduced-sodium soy sauce*
   2 *tbsp catsup*
   2 *tbsp chopped fresh parsley*
   1 *tbsp lemon juice*

    1 clove garlic, minced
    1 tbsp fresh ginger, minced
    6 salmon or swordfish fillets, 5–6 oz each

Mix together all ingredients, except fish. Place fish in 9-inch × 13-inch pan. Pour marinade over fish and marinate in refrigerator 1 hour (or more), turning fish two or three times.

Broil fish, basting with marinade.

SERVES: 6

TANGY DILL SAUCE

    1 cup plain nonfat yogurt
    2 tbsp sour cream
    1 small cucumber, seeded and finely chopped
    2 green onions, thinly sliced
    ½ clove garlic, minced
    ½ tsp dill
    ½ tsp lemon or lime juice

In a small bowl, combine all ingredients and blend well. Cover and chill before serving.

YIELD: 2¼ CUPS

HALIBUT JARDINIERE

    1 cup carrots, julienned
    1 cup celery, julienned
    1 small onion, sliced
    1 tsp olive oil
    2 tbsp water or white wine
    ½ tsp thyme
    1 tsp basil
    ¼ tsp Lite Salt
    ¼ tsp pepper
    2 lb halibut steaks

In a nonstick skillet, sauté carrots, celery, and onion in olive oil until soft, about 5 minutes. Stir in water (or wine), herbs, salt, and pepper. Simmer, covered, 1 minute. Place fish on vegetables. Cover and simmer until fish flakes easily with a fork, about 8 to 10 minutes per inch of thickness.

SERVES: 4 TO 6

FISH A L'ORANGE

   1½ lb fish fillets (orange roughy, sole, cod)
       salt-free seasoning (e.g., Mrs. Dash or Veg-it) **and/or** lemon pepper
    1 tbsp liquid or soft margarine
   1½ tbsp unbleached flour
    ½ cup fresh orange juice
    ¼ cup nonfat milk
    1 tsp grated orange rind
    ½ tsp lemon pepper
    ⅛ tsp nutmeg
    1 green onion, sliced

Place fish fillets in a lightly oiled pan (or use cooking spray). Sprinkle with seasonings. Bake at 400° for 10 minutes per inch of thickness. Turn off oven and leave fish in another 5 to 10 minutes or until it flakes easily with a fork.

Meanwhile, prepare sauce. Melt margarine in a small saucepan. Stir in flour and cook 1 to 2 minutes or until bubbly. Mix orange juice with nonfat milk. Gradually stir into flour; cook and stir until thickened. Add orange rind, lemon pepper, nutmeg, and green onion.

Serve fish immediately topped with 1 to 2 tablespoons of sauce.

SERVES: 6

SNAPPER IN TOMATO-WINE SAUCE

½ onion, chopped
1 cup sliced mushrooms
1 tbsp olive oil
½ cup salt-free tomato sauce
¼ cup dry white wine
½ tsp **each** oregano and basil
2 lb red snapper

Sauté onion and mushrooms in oil. Add tomato sauce, wine, oregano, and basil. Simmer 5 minutes. Place fish in a baking dish coated with cooking spray. Pour sauce over fish. Bake at 350° for 20 to 30 minutes or until fish flakes easily with a fork.

SERVES: 4 TO 6

VEGETABLES

SPICED GREEN BEANS

½ lb fresh green beans
2 tbsp dill seed
1½ cup water
½ cup red wine vinegar
2 tbsp sugar
1 clove garlic, minced
½ tsp celery seed
¼ tsp crushed red pepper
½ cup onion rings

Trim ends from green beans and cut in 2-inch pieces. Place dill seed in a small bowl and crush with a spoon.

In a medium saucepan combine all ingredients except greenbeans and onion. Bring to a boil. Reduce heat and simmer, covered, 5 minutes. Add green beans and onions; simmer until beans are just tender, 2 to 3 minutes.

Pour into a tightly covered container and chill before serving. Add to a tossed salad or serve as an appetizer.

YIELD: 2 TO 3 CUPS

BAKED POTATO TOPPINGS

Instead of the usual high-fat toppings, try:

- HealthMark sour cream (page 204). Add 1 tablespoon chives or thinly sliced green onion

- plain nonfat yogurt mixed with mustard, chives, chopped green onion, dill, parsley, oregano, basil, or horseradish

- chive-yogurt topping: Combine 1 cup plain nonfat yogurt, 2 tablespoons chives or chopped green onion, 1 table-spoon lemon juice, 1 teaspoon grated lemon peel, and 1 clove garlic, minced

- mustard

- lemon juice

- balsamic or other flavored vinegar (a teaspoon or so will be enough)

- barbecue sauce, reduced-sodium catsup; cocktail sauce (just a spoonful or so)

- nonfat cottage cheese

- a few drops **each** sesame oil (dark) and low-sodium soy sauce

- salsa (page 207)

- guacamole

- vegetarian baked beans or vegetarian chili

- 1 tablespoon part-skim Parmesan cheese

OVEN-FRIED POTATOES

2 *baking potatoes, scrubbed*
2 *tsp safflower oil*
¼ *tsp* **each** *salt, pepper, and garlic powder*
½ *tsp paprika*

Slice potatoes into thin strips as for french fries. Toss with oil in a medium bowl. Combine seasonings and sprinkle over potato strips, mixing well.

Spread on nonstick baking sheet. Bake at 350° for 20 to 30 minutes or until browned.

SERVES: 2 TO 4

variation:

Eliminate above seasonings. Sprinkle with herb salt before baking:

herb salt:
1 *tsp salt*
2–3 *tsp garlic powder*
2 *tsp paprika*
1–2 *tsp chili powder*
1 *tsp* **each** *turmeric and pepper*
½ *tsp* **each** *ground ginger, dry mustard, celery seed, onion powder, and dill*

STUFFED BAKED POTATO

6 *potatoes, baked*
1½ *cups HealthMark sour cream (page 204)*
4 *green onions, thinly sliced*
6 *tsp part-skim Parmesan cheese*
paprika

Scoop pulp out of potatoes. Mash and mix with HealthMark sour cream and green onions. Spoon back into potato shells, mounding slightly. Dust tops with cheese and paprika. Bake at 425° until lightly browned, 5 to 10 minutes.

SERVES: 6

RATATOUILLE

      2 cloves garlic, minced
      2 onions, thinly sliced
  1–2 tbsp olive oil
      2 green and/or red peppers, julienned
      2 zucchini, sliced
      1 unpeeled eggplant, chopped
      4 ripe tomatoes, cored and chopped
   ½ tsp **each** salt, pepper, oregano, and basil
   ¼ tsp thyme
      2 tbsp chopped fresh parsley

Sauté garlic and onion in oil until soft. Stir in peppers, zucchini, and eggplant. Continue cooking for 5 minutes, stirring occasionally. Add tomatoes and seasonings. Cover and simmer 20 to 30 minutes, stirring occasionally. Uncover and cook over low heat for 10 to 15 minutes or until liquid evaporates.

SERVES: 8

TOMATOES ROCKEFELLER

      2 tbsp chopped onion
      2 tbsp chopped fresh parsley
   ½ tsp dried savory
  1½ cups cooked, chopped spinach, drained well
      3 ripe tomatoes, halved and seeded
      2 tbsp seasoned bread crumbs
      1 tbsp part-skim Parmesan cheese

Combine onion, parsley, savory, and spinach. Stuff tomatoes with spinach mixture. Mix bread crumbs with cheese and spread on top of tomatoes. Bake at 375° for 15 minutes.

SERVES: 6

BREADS

BRAN MUFFINS

2 cups bran cereal
1 cup nonfat milk
2 egg whites
¼ cup safflower oil
1 cup whole wheat flour
¼ cup brown sugar
2 tsp baking powder
½ cup raisins

Soak cereal in nonfat milk for 1 to 2 minutes to soften. Mix in egg whites and oil.

Sift together flour, sugar, and baking powder in a mixing bowl. Make a well in the center. Add the cereal mixture and raisins. Stir just until flour mixture is moistened. (Do not overmix or muffins will be tough.)

Spoon batter into lightly oiled muffin cups, filling ¾ full. Bake at 425° for 20 to 25 minutes, or until golden brown.

variations:

- Add ½ cup chopped dried apricots, prunes, or blueberries (well drained) to dry ingredients.

- Eliminate bran cereal. Soak 1 cup rolled oats in 1 cup nonfat milk for 15 minutes. Blend with egg whites and oil; add to dry ingredients.

YIELD: 10 TO 12 MUFFINS

ORANGE-OATMEAL MUFFINS

2 tbsp brown sugar
2 tsp whole wheat flour
1 tsp liquid margarine
1/4 tsp cinnamon

1 cup whole wheat flour
1 cup oatmeal, uncooked
1/4 cup chopped pecans
1/4 cup brown sugar
2 tsp grated orange peel
2 tsp baking powder
1/2 cup orange juice
1/4 cup nonfat milk
3 tbsp safflower oil
2 egg whites

Combine first four ingredients; mix until crumbly. Set aside.

Combine 1 cup flour, oatmeal, pecans, sugar, orange rind, and baking powder. Make a well in the center of the mixture. Combine juice, milk, oil, and egg whites. Add to dry ingredients; stir just until moistened.

Spoon mixture into lightly oiled muffin cups, filling three-quarters full. Sprinkle with topping and bake at 425° for 15 minutes.

YIELD: 12 MUFFINS

YOGURT-OAT BRAN MUFFINS

2/3 cup oat bran cereal, uncooked
2/3 cup unbleached flour
1/2 cup whole wheat flour
1/4 cup brown sugar
2 tsp baking powder
1 tsp cinnamon
1/4 tsp cloves

4 *egg whites*
⅔ *cup plain nonfat yogurt*
¼ *cup safflower oil*
½ *cup raisins* **or** *chopped dried fruit (optional)*

Combine oat bran, flours, sugar, baking powder, and spices. Mix egg whites with yogurt and oil. Blend wet and dry ingredients together until just combined.

Fill lightly oiled muffin cups three-quarters full. Bake at 425° for 18 to 20 minutes.

Yield: 12 muffins

BASIC QUICK BREAD

Try any—or all—of the four delicious variations below.

1½ *cups whole wheat flour*
½ *cup oat bran cereal, uncooked*
   leavening (L)
   spice (S)
½ *cup safflower oil*
½ *cup brown sugar*
4 *egg whites*
2 *tsp vanilla*
   fruit (F)

applesauce bread:

L: *1 tsp baking soda*
S: *1 tsp cinnamon*
   ¼ *tsp* **each** *nutmeg and cloves*
F: ¾ *cup unsweetened applesauce*

banana bread:

L: *1 tsp baking soda*
S: *1 tsp* **each** *cinnamon and cardamom*
F: *2 mashed bananas*

pumpkin bread:

L: ½ tsp **each** baking powder and baking soda
S: ½ tsp **each** cloves and cinnamon
¼ tsp nutmeg
F: 1 cup pumpkin

zucchini bread:

L: ½ tsp **each** baking powder and baking soda
S: 1 tsp cinnamon
¼ tsp cloves
F: 1 cup grated, unpeeled zucchini

In a large bowl combine flour, oat bran, leavening, and spices. In a separate bowl beat together oil, sugar, and egg whites until fluffy. Add vanilla and fruit; blend well.

Add dry ingredients to fruit mixture and stir until combined. Pour batter into lightly oiled 9-inch × 5-inch loaf pan. Bake at 350° for 65 to 70 minutes or until tester inserted into center comes out clean.

Cool in pan 10 minutes. Remove from pan and cool on rack.

YIELD: ONE 9-INCH × 5-INCH LOAF

CORN BREAD

½ cup **each** unbleached and whole wheat flour
1 cup cornmeal
2½ tsp baking powder
½ tsp salt (may be omitted)
4 egg whites
¼ cup safflower oil
2 tbsp sugar
1¼ cups nonfat milk **or** 1 cup plain nonfat yogurt and ¼–½ cup nonfat milk

In a medium bowl, blend together flours, cornmeal, baking powder, and salt. In a separate bowl beat together egg whites, oil, sugar, and milk. Mix into flour mixture until just blended.

Pour batter into lightly oiled 8-inch × 8-inch square baking pan. Bake at 425° for 20 to 25 minutes. Serve warm.

YIELD: ONE 8-INCH × 8-INCH LOAF

variation:

Jalapeño Cornbread. Omit salt. Add 1 cup whole kernel corn (if canned, salt-free) and 2 to 4 tablespoons chopped jalapeño or green chili pepper to liquid mixture.

DENISE'S DATE LOAF

    4 egg whites
    ½ cup brown sugar
    8 oz dates, chopped
    1 cup boiling water
    ½ cup safflower oil
    2 cups whole wheat flour
    1 tsp ginger
    1 tsp grated orange peel
    1 tsp **each** baking soda and baking powder

Beat egg whites and brown sugar together. Mix dates, boiling water, and oil; blend with sugar and egg white mixture.

Combine dry ingredients. Add egg white mixture to dry ingredients, mixing until just combined. Turn batter into a lightly oiled 9-inch × 5-inch loaf pan.

Bake at 350° for 1 hour.

YIELD: ONE 9-INCH × 5-INCH LOAF

HEARTY FRUIT AND NUT BREAD

1½ cups unbleached flour
1¼ cups whole wheat flour
¼ cup wheat germ
2½ tsp baking powder
1½ tsp cinnamon
¼ tsp nutmeg
1⅓ cups nonfat milk
½ cup honey **or** brown sugar
¼ cup safflower oil
2 egg whites
1 cup raisins **or** ½ cup **each** raisins and chopped walnuts
¼ cup chopped dates
¼ cup chopped nuts (eliminate if ½ cup walnuts used)

Mix together first six ingredients. Beat milk, honey (or brown sugar), oil, and egg whites together until light and frothy. Stir fruit and nuts into flour mixture. Add milk mixture and stir just until blended. Pour into lightly oiled 9-inch × 5-inch loaf pan. Bake at 325° about 1 hour, or until golden brown.

YIELD: ONE 9-INCH × 5-INCH LOAF

D E S S E R T S

ELLIE'S BROWNIES

⅔ cup safflower oil
1 cup sugar
1½ tsp vanilla
6 egg whites, lightly beaten
¾ cup unbleached flour

½ cup unsweetened cocoa powder
½ tsp baking powder
  pinch salt

Beat together oil, sugar, and vanilla. Add egg whites and mix well. Combine dry ingredients and add to oil mixture, mixing well.

Turn batter into a lightly oiled 8-inch or 9-inch square baking pan. Bake at 350° for 40 to 45 minutes.

When cool, wrap tightly in foil to prevent drying out.

YIELD: 16 BARS

APPLE CRISP

  2 tbsp **each** safflower oil and honey
2½ cups oatmeal, uncooked
  ¼ cup whole wheat flour
  2 tsp cinnamon
  1 tsp allspice
  ½ tsp nutmeg
 10 cooking apples, peeled and sliced
1½ cups raisins
  1 tbsp lemon juice
  2 tsp vanilla
  ½ cup apple **or** orange juice (more if needed)

Combine oil with honey. Mix together with oatmeal, flour, 1 teaspoon cinnamon, ½ teaspoon allspice, and ¼ teaspoon nutmeg. Mix apple slices with raisins, lemon juice, vanilla, and remaining spices.

Lightly oil a 9-inch × 13-inch baking pan. Spread half of the apple mixture in the pan; top with half of the oat mixture. Repeat. Pour on the apple or orange juice. Bake at 325° for 45 minutes, or until topping is crisp.

SERVES: 6 TO 8

OATMEAL COOKIES

⅔ cup soft margarine
⅔ cup brown sugar
2 egg whites
1 tsp vanilla
1⅓ cups unbleached flour **or**
    1 cup unbleached flour plus ⅓ cup whole wheat flour
¼ cup oat bran, uncooked
½ tsp **each** baking soda and cinnamon
¼ tsp nutmeg
2 cups oatmeal, uncooked

Cream margarine and brown sugar in a large bowl. Beat in egg whites and vanilla.

Mix together flour, oat bran, soda, and spices. Gradually add dry ingredients to creamed mixture, mixing well after each addition. (May add up to ¼ cup water or nonfat milk if batter is too thick.) Stir in oatmeal. Drop by teaspoonfuls onto an ungreased cookie sheet 1½ inches apart. Bake at 375° for 12 to 15 minutes.

YIELD: 5 TO 6 DOZEN

HEALTHMARK PUMPKIN PIE

1 16-oz can pumpkin
1 13-oz can evaporated nonfat milk
3 egg whites
½ cup brown sugar
1 tsp vanilla
1 tsp cinnamon
½ tsp nutmeg
¼ tsp cloves
1 9-in graham cracker crust, unbaked (below)

Combine all ingredients and beat well. Pour into unbaked crust and bake at 375° for 50 to 60 minutes.

SERVES: 12

GRAHAM CRACKER CRUST

1¼ cups graham cracker crumbs (Mi-del or Health Valley)
  2 tbsp liquid margarine
 ⅛ tsp nutmeg **or** ½ tsp grated orange peel

Combine ingredients and mix well. Press onto bottom and sides of a 9-inch pie pan. Bake at 375° for 10 minutes.

ANGEL FOOD CAKE

  1 cup sugar
12 egg whites (1½ cups), divided
⅔ cup boiling water
  1 tsp almond extract
½ cup safflower oil
1½ cups unbleached flour
2½ tsp baking powder
½ tsp cream of tartar

Process sugar in food processor until finely ground. Remove and divide in half.

Place ½ cup egg whites, water, extract, and oil in work bowl and process for 2 minutes.

Sift flour, baking powder, and ½ cup sugar. Add to work bowl and process 4 minutes.

Meanwhile in a large bowl, beat remaining 1 cup egg whites until frothy. Add cream of tartar and beat until stiff, then gradually beat in remaining ½ cup sugar, to form a meringue.

Fold flour mixture into meringue until well combined. Pour batter into an ungreased angel food cake pan and bake at 350° for 50 minutes.

Invert pan over a bottle and cool completely before removing cake from pan.

Serve with Basic Fruit Sauce (page 250) or sliced fresh fruit.

INSTANT SORBET

A terrific dessert—ready in an instant

1 20-oz can pineapple, packed in juice, frozen
3 nectarines or peaches
1 cup strawberries, fresh or frozen

Thaw pineapple enough to remove it from the can; cut into chunks. Put in food processor or blender along with other fruit. Process until pureed.

Spread mixture into an 8-inch × 8-inch pan and freeze solid. Thaw enough to break into chunks. Process again in food processor or blender. Freeze mixture until firm.

SERVES: 6

variations:

- Use seasonal fruit of your choice.

- Add 1 cup plain nonfat yogurt and 1 to 2 tablespoons brown sugar **or** 2 to 3 packages Equal to pureed fruit. Amount of sweetener used depends on ripeness of the fruit. Use as little as possible.

BAKED PEARS

2 fresh Bartlett pears
½ cup orange juice
1 tbsp raisins
¼ tsp grated orange peel
1 tsp cornstarch
*　dash allspice*
¼ tsp cinnamon

Cut pears in half lengthwise and core. Pierce inside of pear halves with a fork. Arrange cut side up in a baking dish.

Combine orange juice, raisins, orange peel, cornstarch, and

spices. Cook over medium heat, stirring frequently, until thickened. Pour glaze over pear halves.

Bake at 325° for 20 to 30 minutes or until easily pierced with a fork. Baste several times with glaze during cooking.

SERVES: 4

YOGURT TOPPING

Wonderful on fresh fruit

> 1 *cup plain nonfat yogurt*
> 1–2 *tsp brown sugar, honey,* **or** *2 pkg Equal*
> 1 *tsp vanilla, orange,* **or** *lemon extract*
> 2 *tsp chopped fresh mint (optional)*

Blend all ingredients and chill before serving.

YIELD: 1 CUP

BREAKFASTS

EGG SUBSTITUTE

> 2 *egg whites*
> 1 *tbsp nonfat dry milk*
> 1 *tsp safflower oil*
>   *pinch turmeric (for color, if desired)*

Blend ingredients in a blender until smooth. May be used in baking or for scrambled eggs and omelettes.

YIELD: EQUIVALENT OF 1 EGG

GREEN CHILI OMELETTE

> egg substitute equal to 2 eggs (see page 247)
> 1 tbsp (more or less, to taste) chopped green chili
> 1 corn tortilla
> 2–3 tbsp vegetarian refried beans or black beans
> 1–2 tbsp grated part-skim mozzarella or part-skim Parmesan (optional)
> salsa (page 207)

Beat together egg substitute and green chiles. Pour into a nonstick skillet and cook over low heat until omelette is half done. Top with tortilla, beans, and cheese. Cover pan and cook 1 to 2 minutes more or until omelette is done and beans are heated through (or cheese is melted).

Fold over and slide onto a plate. Top with salsa.

SERVES: 1

OATMEAL PANCAKES

> 2 egg whites
> 1¼ cups buttermilk
> 1 tbsp brown sugar **or** honey
> 2 tbsp safflower oil
> ½ cup oatmeal, uncooked
> ⅔ cup whole wheat flour
> 2 tbsp wheat germ
> ½ tsp baking soda

Beat together egg whites, buttermilk, brown sugar (or honey), and oil. Add dry ingredients. If necessary, thin slightly with 1 to 2 tablespoons nonfat milk.

Pour ¼ cup of batter onto a lightly oiled or nonstick griddle. Cook over moderate heat until tops begin to bubble and edges are dry. Turn and cook until golden brown.

YIELD: TEN TO TWELVE 4-INCH PANCAKES

SUNDAY MORNING PANCAKES

   1 *cup whole wheat flour*
   1 *tsp brown sugar* **or** *honey*
  ½ *tsp baking soda*
   2 *egg whites*
   1 *cup buttermilk or plain nonfat yogurt*
   1 *tbsp safflower oil*

Mix together dry ingredients. Beat together liquid ingredients and add to dry mixture, stirring until blended.

Pour ¼ cup batter onto a lightly oiled nonstick griddle or pan. Cook until bubbly on top and edges are dry. Turn and cook 1 to 2 minutes more, or until golden brown.

YIELD: ABOUT TWELVE 4-INCH PANCAKES

WAFFLES

   3 *egg whites*
   2 *cups buttermilk*
   1 *cup unbleached flour*
   1 *cup whole wheat flour*
  ¼ *cup wheat germ*
   2 *tsp baking powder*
   1 *tsp baking soda*
   1 *tsp vanilla*
  ⅓ *cup safflower oil*

Heat waffle iron. Lightly beat egg whites until frothy; fold in remaining ingredients until smooth.

Pour batter into center of hot waffle iron. Bake about 5 minutes or until waffle stops steaming. **Note:** Do not overbake or waffles will be dry.

YIELD: EIGHT 7-INCH WAFFLES

BASIC FRUIT SAUCE

Use on pancakes, french toast, waffles, or as a topping for yogurt or angel food cake.

> 2 *cups apple juice*
> 1 *tbsp cornstarch*
> 1 *tsp vanilla*

Blend apple juice gradually with cornstarch; cook over medium heat, stirring frequently, until thickened, 4 to 5 minutes. Add vanilla and fruit.

blueberry sauce: Add 1 cup blueberries.
strawberry sauce: Add 1 cup sliced strawberries.
apple sauce: Add 2 peeled and chopped apples and 1 teaspoon cinnamon; simmer until apples are soft.
orange sauce: Add 1 cup orange segments and 1 teaspoon grated orange peel.

YIELD: 2 CUPS

GRANOLA

> 4 *cups oatmeal, uncooked*
> ½ *cup* **each** *wheat germ and bran*
> ½ *cup chopped unsalted, dry roasted nuts* **or**
>   ½ *cup unsalted dry roasted sunflower seeds* **or** *a combination of both*
> 1½ *tsp cinnamon*
> ¼ *cup honey*
> ¼ *cup safflower oil*
> ⅔ *cup raisins* **or** *other dried fruit*

Combine oats, wheat germ, bran, nuts, and cinnamon. Heat honey and oil together, stirring until well blended (or heat in microwave about 1 minute, stirring until blended). Pour over oat mixture and mix well.

Spread onto baking pan. Bake at 350° for 25 to 30 minutes or until slightly browned, stirring occasionally.

to prepare in microwave:

Cook on HIGH for 8 to 10 minutes, stirring every 2 minutes. Cool, then stir in raisins. Store in airtight container.

YIELD: ABOUT 6 CUPS

BAKED APPLES

4 *small apples, cored*
½ *cup apple juice*
2 *tbsp raisins*
cinnamon and nutmeg
½ *cup water*

Place apples in a baking dish. Fill each cavity with 1 tablespoon apple juice, and 1½ teaspoons raisins. Sprinkle with cinnamon and nutmeg.

Pour remaining apple juice and water into baking dish. Bake at 350° until soft.

SERVES: 4

Index

253